ACKNOWLEDGMENTS

Many people have contributed to this book and we sincerely thank them all. Catherine Saxelby, consultant dietitian, got us off to a good start, then cast her expert eye over the final manuscript; publisher Philippa Sandall put her faith in us, and brought the book to fruition; Alison Saunders expertly tested the recipes to ensure their success; many nutrition students and volunteers from the Human Nutrition Unit of the University of Sydney undertook G.I. testing of many foods; PhD students, Susanne Holt and Diana Thomas, masterminded the satiety and sports performance studies and Kellogg Australia generously funded their research; Isa Hopwood typed up the list of G.I. factors and the index; dietitians Rudi Bartl, Helen O'Connor and Martina Chippendall contributed to various chapters; and lastly, we thank our long-suffering spouses, John Miller, Jacqueline Leeds, Jonathan Powell and Ruth Colagiuri, respectively, for their sense of humour and unswerving (well, most of the time) support.

For the UK edition, the book was reviewed and the recipes tested by many people. Catherine Bryan, SRD, advised on the content from a UK dietitian's point of view and developed new recipes assisted by Jackie Green, SRD. Mary Moloney of the Dublin Institute of Technology reviewed the text and gave guidance from an Irish perspective. Alexandra Becket and Charlotte Townsend of King's College London kindly provided secretarial support, and Rowena Webb and Laura Brockbank managed the project with forbearance for the publisher. The authors are grateful for the help so given.

The Glucose Revolution

The groundbreaking medical discovery of the G.I. factor for

WEIGHT LOSS
PEAK SPORTS PERFORMANCE
BLOOD SUGAR CONTROL
REDUCING THE RISK OF HEART DISEASE

Dr Anthony Leeds
Associate Professor Jennie Brand-Miller
Kaye Foster-Powell
Dr Stephen Colagiuri

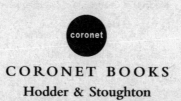

CORONET BOOKS
Hodder & Stoughton

First published as *The G.I. Factor* in Australia in 1996 by
Hodder and Stoughton (Australia) Pty Ltd

First published as *The G.I. Factor* in Great Britain in 1996 by
arrangement with Hodder and Stoughton (Australia) Pty Ltd

First published in Great Britain in 2000 by Hodder and Stoughton
First published in paperback in 2001 by Hodder and Stoughton
A division of Hodder Headline

A Coronet Paperback

10 9 8 7 6 5 4 3 2

A CIP catalogue record for this title
is available from the British Library.

ISBN 0 340 76826 6

Printed and bound in Great Britain by
Mackays of Chatham PLC, Chatham, Kent

Hodder and Stoughton
A division of Hodder Headline
338 Euston Road
London NW1 3BH

ABOUT THE AUTHORS

ASSOCIATE PROFESSOR JENNIE BRAND MILLER is a member of the teaching and research staff of the Human Nutrition Unit, Department of Biochemistry, University of Sydney. She graduated BSc (1975) and PhD (1979) from the Department of Food Science and Technology at the University of New South Wales. She has more than one hundred and fifty publications to her name, including fifty on the glycaemic index of foods and its applications to diabetes, sport and satiety.

DR ANTHONY LEEDS is senior lecturer in the Department of Nutrition and Dietetics at King's College London. He graduated in medicine from the Middlesex Hospital Medical School in 1971. He was a fellow clinical student with David Jenkins (who described the glycaemic index in 1981) from 1968 and worked with him at the Medical Research Council Gastroenterology Unit until 1977. He continues to research on carbohydrate and dietary fibre in relation to high blood cholesterol, obesity and diabetes, continues part-time medical practice, and is a member of the European Association of Scientific Editors. He chairs the Forum on Food and Health at the Royal Society of Medicine, the Accreditation Committee of the Institute of Biologists' Register of Nutritionists, and the Research Ethics Committee of King's College London.

KAYE FOSTER-POWELL is an accredited practising dietitian-nutritionist. In 1987 she graduated BSc (Honours) and completed a Masters of Nutrition and Dietetics (1994), both from the University of Sydney. She has extensive experience in diabetes management and has researched practical applications of the glycaemic index over the last five years. Currently she is the senior dietitian at Wentworth Area Diabetes Service and conducts a private practice in the Blue Mountains, New South Wales.

ASSOCIATE PROFESSOR STEPHEN COLAGIURI is the Director of the Diabetes Centre and Head of the Department of Endocrinology, Metabolism and Diabetes at the Prince of Wales Hospital in Randwick, New South Wales. He graduated MBBS from the University of Sydney in 1970 and received his Fellowship of the Royal Australasian College of Physicians in 1977. He has an appointment as Senior Lecturer at the University of New South Wales. He has over one hundred scientific papers to his name, many concerned with the importance of carbohydrate in the diet of people with diabetes.

CONTENTS

DISPELLING SOME MYTHS ABOUT FOOD

This book dispels many myths about food and carbohydrate.

We now know from our scientific research into the glycaemic index that the following popular beliefs about food and carbohydrate are not true.

MYTH 1   **Starchy foods like bread and potatoes are fattening.**
Not true, bread and potatoes are carbohydrate foods and therefore among the best foods you can eat to help you lose weight.

MYTH 2   **Sugar is the worst thing for people with diabetes.**
Not true, sugar, even eaten alone, has no greater effect on blood sugar levels than most starchy foods. Fat is the worst thing for people with diabetes.

MYTH 3   **All starches are slowly digested in the intestine.**
Not true, some starch, like that in potatoes, is digested in a flash.

MYTH 4   **Sugar causes high blood pressure.**
Not true, sugar has no direct effect on blood pressure. Salt and salty foods increase blood pressure in those at risk.

MYTH 5   **Hunger pangs are inevitable if you want to lose weight.**
Not true, high carbohydrate foods, especially those with a low G.I. factor (e.g. rolled oats and pasta), will sustain the feeling of fullness almost to the next meal.

MYTH 6   **Sugar is fattening.**
Not true, sugar has no special fattening properties. It is no more likely to be turned into fat than any other carbohydrate. Sugar, which is often present in foods with concentrated energy and fat, may sometimes seem to be 'turned to fat', but it's the total energy (calories) rather than the sugar in those energy dense foods that causes more fat to be made.

MYTH 7   **Starches are best for optimum sports performance.**
Not true, in many instances starchy foods are too bulky to eat in the quantities needed for active sports people.

MYTH 8   **Foods high in fat are more filling.**
Not true, recent studies show that high fat foods are among the least filling. It is extremely easy to 'passively overconsume' foods like potato chips and crisps.

MYTH 9   **Diets high in sugar are less nutritious.**
Not true, studies have shown that diets high in sugar (from a range of sources including dairy food and fruit) often have higher levels of micronutrients such as calcium, riboflavin and vitamin C.

MYTH 10   **High fat diets are always high in sugar.**
Not true, the reality is that high fat diets can be low in sugar and vice versa. Most sources of fat in the diet are not sweetened (e.g. potato chips) and most sources of sugar contain no fat (e.g. soft drinks).

KEY POINTS FROM THE GLYCAEMIC INDEX (G.I.) FACTOR

- The modern diet is too high in fat and not high enough in carbohydrate.

- The carbohydrate we eat is digested and absorbed too quickly because most modern starchy foods have a high G.I. factor.

- The G.I. Factor is a ranking of foods based on their over-all effect on blood sugar levels (low G.I. means a smaller rise of blood sugar).

- Middle-aged people who follow a low G.I. diet may be less likely to develop diabetes.

- Low G.I. diets can help control established diabetes.

- Low G.I. diets can help people lose weight.

- Low G.I. diets may help lower blood lipids.

- Low G.I. diets can improve the body's sensitivity to insulin.

- Low G.I. diets may help reduce the risk of heart disease in some people.

- Low G.I. foods reduce the G.I. of the meal as a whole.

- A high G.I. factor food + a low G.I. factor food = an inter-mediate G.I. factor meal.

- To make the change use more:

  - low G.I. breakfast cereals (based on wheatbran and oats)

  - whole grain breads (especially using barley and rye)

  - pasta products in place of potatoes

  - low G.I. fruits: pears, plums, apples

- Think less about simple and complex carbohydrate.

  - **Think low G.I.**

INTRODUCTION

•

The right kind of carbohydrate can make an important contribution to the quality of your life. This book about the glycaemic index, what we have called the G.I. factor, will help you choose the right amount of carbohydrate and the right sort of carbohydrate for your lifestyle and your wellbeing. It will help you increase your food intake without increasing your waistline. If you don't use the G.I. factor to improve your body balance or your sports performance, then you will be missing out.

The G.I. factor is a scientifically validated tool in the dietary management of diabetes, weight reduction and athletic performance. Foods with a **low G.I. factor** help people control their hunger, their appetite and their blood sugar levels. These foods actually help athletes prolong endurance when eaten before an event. After the first event, foods with a **high G.I. factor** have been shown to replenish energy stores faster and give athletes greater staying power for further events.

The G.I. factor (glycaemic index) of foods is simply a ranking of foods based on their immediate effect on blood sugar levels.

■ Carbohydrate foods that break down quickly during digestion have the highest G.I. factors. Their blood sugar response is fast and high.

■ Carbohydrates which break down slowly, releasing glucose gradually into the bloodstream, have low G.I. factors.

■■■■ THE GOOD NEWS

Our research on the G.I. factor began in the 1980s when health authorities all over the world began to stress the importance of high carbohydrate diets. Until then dietary fat had grabbed all the media attention (and to some extent this is still true). But low-fat diets are *ipso facto* high in carbohydrate. The questions became which type of carbohydrate is best for:

- good health,
- people who play sport, and
- people with diabetes?

Our research since the early 1980s has contributed to the worldwide recognition that the rate of carbohydrate digestion in the gastro-intestinal (digestive) tract has important implications for everybody.

Although the G.I. factor has been well described in scientific journals and nutrition text books over the past decade, the information was locked away in the scientific literature. We believe that it is time to spread the good news to a wider audience and to broadcast the fact that there are different types of carbohydrate that work in different ways. So, we wrote this book to give you a guide to the physiological effects of a food on your blood sugar levels.

The good news is that the G.I. factor provides an easier and more effective way to win the battle of the bulge and control fluctuations in blood sugar (glucose). People with diabetes in the family and serious athletes will welcome the news. For some people it will lift the great burden of guilt about eating. This is the first book to bring you the facts about carbohydrate and the G.I. factor.

■■■ WHO IS THIS BOOK FOR?

The Glucose Revolution is for just about everybody. In particular it is for people who will gain most from putting the G.I. factor approach into practice — people with diabetes, athletes, and people who are overweight. Most people have some notion of how blood sugar rises and falls. However, much of the information currently in print about food and blood sugar is wrong. *The Glucose Revolution* gives you the true story about carbohydrate and the blood sugar connection.

This book gives people with diabetes a new lease of life, literally! Many people with diabetes find that despite doing all the right things, their blood sugar levels remain too high. The G.I. factor allows people with diabetes to choose the right kind of carbohydrate for blood sugar control.

This book gives athletes the competitive edge over their rivals by allowing them to choose the right carbohydrate for optimum sports performance. Some athletes already know something about carbohydrate loading but think that it sounds too complicated. Others are now following a high carbohydrate diet but wonder whether some types of carbohydrate are better than others.

This book also helps answer the questions about sugar from worried parents who are concerned about their family's health and wellbeing.

▬▬▬ HOW YOU CAN USE THIS BOOK

Please don't be tempted to skip the early chapters of this book and jump straight into the specific applications of the G.I. factor for weight loss, diabetes or sports performance. We recommend you read the introductory chapters as they will give you a complete overview of the carbohydrate story. The facts we reveal about carbohydrate will surprise many people — facts that can make life a lot easier.

Part I contains the most up-to-date information about what makes a balanced diet and why — information based on scientific research, clinical trials and real-life experiences. It stresses the value of a high carbohydrate and low-fat diet for everybody. It tells you which types of carbohydrate are best and why. It explains why the G.I. factor is the best tool for choosing the right types of carbohydrate for your needs and your lifestyle. Chapters cover how you can use the G.I. factor to lose weight, lower blood sugar levels, improve sports performance, and possibly reduce the risk of heart disease.

In Part II we show you how you can include more of the right sort of carbohydrate in your diet, give hints for meal preparation, and practical tips and food combinations to help you to make the G.I. factor work for you throughout the day. This section includes over fifty imaginative and delicious recipes for breakfast, lunch, dinner and in-between snacks which we have developed and tested along with their G.I. factor and nutritional analysis.

If it's just the G.I. factors you are after, you'll find them in Part III which contains an A to Z listing over 250 foods and their G.I. factors. Finally there's a list of scientific references on pages 224 to 226 to back up all we say.

Jennie Brand Miller   Anthony Leeds
Kaye Foster-Powell
Stephen Colagiuri   London 2000

Sydney 2000

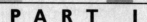

PART I

WHAT YOU NEED TO KNOW ABOUT THE G.I. FACTOR

WHAT'S WRONG WITH TODAY'S DIET?

WHAT OUR ANCESTORS ATE

WHAT WE REALLY NEED TO EAT
FOR HEALTH AND GROWTH

WHAT'S WRONG WITH TODAY'S DIET?

WITH A WAVE OF THE FAT WAND

WHY WE NEED TO EAT MORE CARBOHYDRATE

SO, WHAT IS A BALANCED DIET?

●

▬▬ WHAT OUR ANCESTORS ATE

For 10 000 years, our ancestors survived on a high carbohydrate and low-fat diet. They ate their carbohydrate in the form of beans, vegetables and whole cereal grains. They ate their sugars in fibrous fruits and berries. Food preparation was a simple process: grinding food between stones and cooking it over the heat of an open fire. The result of this process was that all food was digested and absorbed slowly and the usual blood sugar rise was gradual and prolonged. This was ideal as far as their bodies were concerned because it provided slow-release energy that helped to delay hunger pangs and provided fuel for working muscles long after the meal was eaten. It was also kind to their pancreas.

THE PANCREAS

The pancreas is a vital organ near the stomach. Its job is to produce the hormone insulin. Carbohydrate stimulates the secretion of insulin more than any other component of food. The slow absorption of the carbohydrate in our food means that the pancreas doesn't have to work so hard and produces less insulin.

As time passed, the flours were ground more and more finely and the bran was separated completely from the white flour. With the advent of high speed roller mills in the nineteenth century, it was possible to produce white flour so fine that it resembled talcum powder in appearance and texture. These fine white flours have always been highly prized because they make soft bread and delicious, fluffy sponge cakes. Fruit varieties such as apples and oranges were also selected because of their higher sweetness and lower fibre content. As incomes grew, the legumes and beans commonly eaten by our grandparents were cast aside and meat consumption increased. As a consequence, the composition of the average diet changed: we began to eat more fat and the type of carbohydrate in our diet changed, becoming more quickly digested and absorbed. Something we didn't expect happened, too. The blood sugar rise after a meal was higher and more prolonged, stimulating the pancreas to produce more insulin.

So not only did we have higher blood sugar levels after a meal, we had higher insulin responses as well. Insulin is a hormone that is needed for carbohydrate metabolism. But it has a profound effect on the development of many diseases. Medical experts now believe that high insulin levels are one of the key factors responsible for heart disease and hypertension. Insulin influences the way we metabolise foods, determining whether we burn fat or carbohydrate to meet our energy needs and ultimately determining whether we store fat in our body.

Thus one of the most important ways in which our diet differs from that of our ancestors is the **speed of carbohydrate digestion and the resulting effect on blood sugar and insulin levels**. In summary, traditional diets all around the world contained slowly digested and absorbed carbohydrate — foods that we now know have a **low** G.I. factor (glycaemic index). In contrast, modern diets with their quickly digested fine white flours are based on foods with a **high** G.I. factor (glycaemic index).

▬▬▬ WHAT WE REALLY NEED TO EAT FOR HEALTH AND GROWTH

Food is part of our culture and way of life. Our food choices are determined by many factors ranging from religious beliefs to the deliciously sensual role that food plays in our lives. For babies, food has a comforting role to play, beyond meeting the immediate physical need. For adults, food reflects status — we prepare special meals for special occasions and for special guests to show respect or friendship.

It is no wonder that with so many factors influencing our food choices, we tend to overlook the very basic role food plays in the nourishment and growth of our bodies. In a busy lifestyle, it's easy to see food simply as a solution to overcoming hunger. In other circumstances we focus on the social aspects of food and eat too much.

In Australia the CSIRO Division of Human Nutrition has developed a pyramid food model to give visual guidance on the types and amounts of foods which should be eaten. In the Republic of Ireland a similar food pyramid is used, while in the United Kingdom the different food groups are presented on a plate model. Differences of detail (e.g. the total number of fruit and vegetable servings — seven in Australia, four in Ireland, five in the UK) reflect differing patterns of food consumption. For many reasons our eating habits fall very short of these recommendations.

Kilocalorie-laden foods and drinks (sometimes called energy dense foods), such as alcohol, chocolate, chips and confectionery, provide few nutrients for a lot of kilocalories. For this reason they are referred to as indulgences and are best limited to no more than two per day.

▬▬▬ WHAT'S WRONG WITH TODAY'S DIET?

Today's Western diet is the product of industrialisation based on inventions ranging from Jethro Tull's seed drill (in 1701) to the high speed steel roller mills for milling cereals (in the nineteenth century) and advances in processing food to give it a longer shelf life. The benefits are many. We have a plentiful, relatively cheap, palatable (some would say too palatable) and safe food supply. Gone are the days of monotonous fare, gaps in the food supply, weevil-infested and adulterated food. Long gone are widespread vitamin deficiencies such as scurvy and pellagra. Today's food manufacturers work hard to bring us irresistible products that meet the demands of both gourmands and health conscious consumers.

Many of the new foods are still based on our staple cereals — fine white cereal flours, particularly wheat flour. High speed roller mills break down the grains to produce a fine flour with small particle size that produces the best quality breads, cakes, biscuits, breakfast cereals and extruded snack foods.

Cereal chemists and bakers know that the finest particle size flour produces the most palatable and shelf-stable end product. But this striving for excellence in one area has resulted in unforeseen problems in another. Today's staple carbohydrate foods, including ordinary bread, are quickly digested and absorbed. The resulting effect on blood sugar levels has created a problem for many of us.

▅▅▅ WITH A WAVE OF THE FAT WAND...

One of the most undesirable aspects of the modern diet is its high fat content. Food manufacturers, bakers and chefs know we love to eat fat. We love its creaminess and mouth feel and find it easy to consume in excess. It makes our meat more tender, our vegetables and salads more palatable and our sweet foods even more desirable. We prefer potatoes as French fries or potato crisps, to have our fish battered and fried and our pastas in rich creamy sauces. With a wave of the fat wand, bland high carbohydrate foods like rice and oats are magically transformed into very palatable, kilocalorie-laden foods such as fried rice and toasted muesli. In fact, when you analyse it, much of our diet today is an undesirable but delicious combination of both fat and quickly digested carbohydrate.

....

WHAT'S WRONG WITH OUR WAY OF EATING?

▓ The modern diet is too high in fat and therefore not high enough in carbohydrate.

▓ The carbohydrate we eat is digested and absorbed too quickly because most modern starchy foods have a high G.I. factor.

....

▆▆▆▆ WHY WE NEED MORE CARBOHYDRATE

For once the experts on health are unanimous. They all agree that the food we eat for breakfast, lunch and dinner and for those in-between snacks should be low in fat and high in carbohydrate. The same diet that helps prevent our becoming overweight also reduces our risk of developing heart disease, diabetes and many types of cancer. This same high carbohydrate and low-fat diet improves sports performance.

But the story doesn't finish there. To reduce the fat content of our diet, we need to eat lots of high carbohydrate, low-fat foods. Carbohydrate should be the main source of energy in our food, not fat. Carbohydrate and fat have a reciprocal relationship in our diet. The more carbohydrate we eat, the lower our fat intake. The new emphasis on eating lots of high carbohydrate foods has focused attention on **the differences between carbohydrates**.

▆▆▆▆ SO, WHAT IS A BALANCED DIET?

It makes sense to balance our food intake with the rate our bodies use it. This way, we maintain a steady weight. These days, however, this balance is difficult to achieve. It is very easy to overeat. Refined foods, convenience foods and fast foods frequently lack fibre and conceal fat so that before we feel full, we have overdosed on kilocalories. It is even easier not to exercise. It takes longer to walk somewhere than it does to drive (except perhaps in the rush hour). With intake exceeding output on a regular basis, the result for too many of us is weight gain.

Times have changed from the days of our hunter-gatherer ancestors. We need to adapt our lifestyle to our more kilocalorie-laden diet and fewer physical demands. It's become very important to **catch** bursts of physical activity wherever we can to increase our energy output. It may mean using the stairs instead of the lift, taking a 10 minute walk at lunch time, coasting on a treadmill while you watch the news, walking to the shops to get the Sunday paper, parking half a mile from work, or taking the dog for a walk each night. Whatever it means, do it. Even housework burns kilocalories. All these seemingly small bursts of activity accumulate to increase our kilocalorie output.

While you work on increasing your kilocalorie output, the G.I. factor can help you select the best foods to balance your intake. Its high carbohydrate basis ensures a filling diet which isn't packed with kilocalories.

So, our first message is reduce the amount of fat you eat. This applies to all sorts of fat: saturated, polyunsaturated, monounsaturated. (While a low-fat diet is good for most of us, it is not appropriate for children who rely on fat for growth.) But the flip side of this message is eat more carbohydrate because this will automatically reduce your fat intake. The following chapters tell you how you can eat more carbohydrate and which foods you should choose to replace fatty foods. It also goes one step further and tells you which carbohydrates are best for health — and why.

CHAPTER 2

THE HIGH CARBOHYDRATE DIET

HOW DOES CARBOHYDRATE WORK?

SO, WHAT MAKES A HIGH CARBOHYDRATE DIET?

HOW MUCH CARBOHYDRATE DO YOU
NEED IN A DAY?

CARBOHYDATE REQUIREMENTS FOR SMALL EATERS

CARBOHYDRATE REQUIREMENTS FOR
BIGGER EATERS

WHAT'S WRONG WITH THIS MENU?

WHAT ABOUT THE DIFFERENT TYPES
OF CARBOHYDRATE?

THE CARBOHYDRATE/G.I. FACTOR LINK

•

Our bodies burn fuel all the time and the fuel our bodies like best is carbohydrate. Just as you would never try to run your car without petrol — its essential energy source — you should not try to run your body without carbohydrate — your body's preferred energy source. Carbohydrate is the fuel we use when we walk, talk, think, move, scratch, sneeze, jump, or sleep. Everything!

You might think of carbohydrate as the all important ingredient that makes foods taste sweet. It is also the starchy part of foods like rice, bread, potatoes and pasta. In fact, carbohydrate is the most widely consumed nutrient in the world, after water. It's important to the human body because it yields glucose. Glucose is so important that if your diet doesn't provide enough carbohydrate, your brain signals a shortage of glucose, and muscle tissue will be broken down to supply the shortfall. This basically means that you lose body muscle to feed your brain. This undesirable state of affairs is strong argument for including the minimum of carbohydrate in your daily diet. Fifty to 60 per cent of your daily kilojoule intake should come from carbohydrate.

■■■■ HOW DOES CARBOHYDRATE WORK?

The ultimate source of glucose for the body is from the sugars and starches in food. To make use of these, the body must first break them down in the gut into a form that can be absorbed and which the cells can use. This process is called digestion.

Digestion starts in the mouth when **amylase**, the digestive enzyme in saliva, is incorporated into the food by chewing. The activity of this enzyme stops in the stomach. Most of the digestion continues only when the carbohydrate reaches the small intestine. In the small intestine, amylase from pancreatic juice breaks down the large molecules of starch into short chain molecules. These and any **disaccharide** sugars are then broken into simpler monosaccharides by enzymes in the wall of the intestine. The **monosaccharides** that result, **glucose, fructose** and **galactose**, are absorbed from the small intestine into the bloodstream where they are available as a source of energy to the cells.

The blood maintains a certain level of glucose to serve the brain and central nervous system. These organs cannot function properly without glucose. To ensure a continual supply of glucose, the body stores its glucose reserves in the muscles and the liver in the form of glycogen. If you are eating insufficient carbohydrate, these glycogen reserves are mobilised and converted to glucose. Once the body has used up its glycogen it will start breaking down muscle protein to synthesise glucose for the vital organs. A low carbohydrate diet will make you feel headachy and unwell and causes loss of lean muscle tissue and water — two things you need to hang onto! It will not help you lose weight because the body's fat stores cannot be converted to glucose.

WHAT IS A CARBOHYDRATE?

Carbohydrate is a part of food. Starch is a carbohydrate, so too are sugars and certain types of fibre. Starches are nature's reserves created by energy from the sun, carbon dioxide and water. The building block of starch is glucose, a single sugar.

The simplest form of carbohydrate is a single sugar molecule. Chemically, this sugar molecule is known as a **monosaccharide** (**mono** meaning one, **saccharide** meaning sweet). Glucose is a single sugar molecule which occurs in foods and is the most common source of fuel for the cells of the human body.

If two sugar molecules are joined together, the result is a **disaccharide** (**di** meaning two). Sucrose, or common table sugar, is a disaccharide.

Starches are long chains of sugar molecules joined together like the beads in a string of pearls. They are called **polysaccharides** (**poly** meaning many). Starches are not sweet to taste.

Dietary fibres also have a complex structure, containing many different sorts of sugar molecules. They are different from starches and sugars in that they are not broken down by human digestive enzymes. Fibre reaches the large intestine without change. Once there, bacteria begin to ferment and break down the fibres.

SUGARS FOUND IN FOOD

Monosaccharides	Disaccharides
(single sugar molecules)	(two single sugar molecules joined together)
glucose	maltose = glucose + glucose
fructose	sucrose = glucose + fructose
galactose	lactose = glucose + galactose

SOURCES OF CARBOHYDRATE

Carbohydrate mainly comes from plant foods, such as cereal grains, fruits, vegetables and legumes (peas and beans). Milk also contains carbohydrate. The following list includes foods that are high in carbohydrate and provide very little fat. Eat lots of them, sparing the butter, margarine and oil during their preparation.

Cereal grains including rice, wheat, oats, barley, rye and anything made from them such as bread, pasta, breakfast cereal, flour.

Fruits including apples, oranges, bananas, grapes, peaches, melons etc.

Vegetables such as potatoes, yams, sweet corn and sweet potato are all high in carbohydrate.

Legumes, peas and **beans** including baked beans, lentils, kidney beans, chick peas etc.

Milk contains carbohydrate too, in the form of milk sugar or lactose. Lactose is the first carbohydrate we encounter as infants. Use semi-skimmed or skimmed milk and yoghurt to minimise fat intake. Many low-fat dairy products contain some sugar. It helps to make these rather bland or acidic foods more palatable. The sugar content of these products is not a problem.

SOURCES OF CARBOHYDRATE

Percentage of carbohydrate in grams per 100 grams of food

apple 12%	grapes 15%	pear 12%	sweet corn 16%
baked beans 11%	ice cream 22%	plum 6%	sweet potato....17%
banana 21%	milk...................5%	potato 15–20%	tapioca 85%
barley...............61%	oats 61%	rice 79%	water biscuit 71%
bread................47%	orange................8%	split peas..........45%	wheat biscuit....62%
cornflakes 85%	pasta.................70%	sugar..............100%	
flour 73%	peas 8%	sultanas 75%	

■■■ SO, WHAT MAKES A HIGH CARBOHYDRATE DIET?

Eating a high carbohydrate diet means:

- ■ eating carbohydrate-rich foods at every meal and making sure that carbohydrates form a large proportion of the meal,
- ■ eating carbohydrate-rich foods for snacks,
- ■ including at least the minimum quantity of carbohydrate foods suggested for small eaters (see page 14).

Eating a high carbohydrate diet also means:

- ■ not eating too much protein or fat. High fat foods are a concentrated source of energy. It takes only a small extra amount of them to throw your diet out of balance.

Remember, if you are eating a high carbohydrate diet then you'll automatically be eating less fat.

■■■ HOW MUCH CARBOHYDRATE DO YOU NEED IN A DAY?

Most of the world's population eat a high carbohydrate diet based on staples such as rice, maize (corn), millet and wheat-based foods like pasta or bread. In developing countries, carbohydrate may form 70 to 80 per cent of a person's energy (kilocalorie) intake. In developed countries the intake may be half this. In the United States and Canada, the United Kingdom, Ireland, Australia and New Zealand, carbohydrate typically contributes only 40 to 45 per cent of energy (kilocalorie) intake. In these countries, carbohydrate, the body's vital energy source, tends to be crowded out by protein and fat.

Current recommendations suggest that we should be taking at least 50 to 55 per cent of our total energy intake as carbohydrate. To do this we need to consume 150 grams of carbohydrate for every 1000 kilocalories (4200 kilojoules). For a low energy diet (1200 kilocalories/5000 kilojoules) it means eating about 190 grams of carbohydrate per day (equivalent to 14 slices of bread). A young, active person with higher energy requirements, say in the order of 2000 kilocalories (8400 kilojoules), would require 300 grams of carbohydrate (equivalent to 24 slices of bread). As an example of what this looks like we have calculated a sample carbohydrate intake for small eaters and bigger eaters (see pages 14 to 15).

The number of kilocalories and hence the amount of carbohydrate needed varies greatly between people. Your kilocalorie requirements depend on your age, sex, activity level and body size. It is not possible to publish standard figures that will apply to every reader. If you want more information on your own specific kilocalorie and carbohydrate needs, we suggest that you consult a dietitian. Dietitians can help you assess your energy requirements and calculate exactly how much carbohydrate you need. Most of us don't need to consult dietitians or keep count of the number of grams of carbohydrate we eat every day. But for some people, like athletes, it may be necessary to keep a watch to make sure that they are eating enough carbohydrate.

HOW TO FIND A DIETITIAN

If you feel that you need to consult a dietitian about your energy requirements and how much carbohydrate you should be eating, consult your family doctor (GP) or contact the British Dietetic Association, 7th Floor, Elizabeth House, 22 Suffolk Street, Queensway, Birmingham, B1 1LS. Make sure that the person you choose is a State Registered Dietitian (in the UK) or a member of the Irish Nutrition and Dietetic Institute (Dundrum Business Centre, Franfort, Dublin 14) designated by SRD or MINDI after the name, respectively.

However, if you are looking at ways to improve your own diet there are three important things to remember:

1. Identify the sources of fat and look at ways you can reduce it or eliminate the high fat food entirely.
2. You may need to eat more when you add more carbohydrate to your diet. Most people do.
3. A low-fat diet is not appropriate for children under 5 years of age. They need the extra energy provided by fat for normal growth and development.

▆▆▆ CARBOHYDRATE REQUIREMENTS FOR SMALL EATERS

You might consider yourself a small eater if you:

- ▆ are a small-framed female,
- ▆ have a small appetite,
- ▆ do very little physical activity,
- ▆ are trying to lose weight.

Even the smallest eater needs these carbohydrate foods every day:

- ▆ around 4 slices of bread or the equivalent (crackers, rolls, English style muffins)
  PLUS
- ▆ about 3 pieces of fruit or the equivalent (juice, dried fruit)
  PLUS
- ▆ 1 large serving of high carbohydrate vegetables (corn, legumes, potato, sweet potato)
  PLUS
- ▆ at least 1 large serving of cereal or grain food (breakfast cereal, cooked rice or pasta, or other grains)
  PLUS
- ▆ 400 ml (14 fl oz) semi-skimmed milk or the equivalent (yoghurt, ice cream). This includes milk in your tea and coffee and with your cereal

If this amount of food sounds right for you, try it as a minimum amount of carbohydrate. This supplies 225 grams of carbohydrate, suitable for a 1500 kilocalorie (6300 kilojoule) diet.

Listen to your appetite if it demands more.

■■■ CARBOHYDRATE REQUIREMENTS
FOR BIGGER EATERS

The picture of a bigger eater would fit you if you are:
■ an active young female of average frame size,
■ doing regular physical activity (but not strenuous exercise),
■ an adult male or teenage boy,
■ working as a labourer.

Bigger eaters need to eat:
■ around 8 slices of bread or the equivalent (crackers, rolls, English style muffins)
  PLUS
■ about 3 pieces of fruit or the equivalent (juice, dried fruit)
  PLUS
■ 2 large servings of high carbohydrate cooked vegetables (corn, legumes, potato, sweet potato)
  PLUS
■ at least 2 large servings of cereal or grain food (breakfast cereal or cooked rice, or pasta or other grain)
  PLUS
■ 400 ml (14 fl oz) semi-skimmed milk or the equivalent (yoghurt, ice cream)

This provides 375 grams of carbohydrate which is suitable for a 2500 kilocalorie (10 500 kilojoule) diet. This is appropriate for a young, active adult of average build.

An athlete who is training hard would generally need to eat double this quantity of carbohydrate.

Carbohydrate is the most satiating of all nutrients. This simply means that it satisfies your appetite and fills you up. Over-consumption of food is highly unlikely on a high carbohydrate and low-fat diet. So, base your diet on high fibre carbohydrate foods like whole grain breads, cereals, fruit, vegetables and legumes and let your appetite dictate how much you need to eat.

▰▰▰ WHAT'S WRONG WITH THIS MENU?

Take a look at this menu. To many people, it may sound very familiar.

- **BREAKFAST**
  2 slices wholemeal toast with butter and yeast extract spread
  white coffee, no sugar

- **MID-MORNING SNACK**
  an apple
  white tea

- **LUNCH**
  a large mixed salad containing a range of vegetables with a slice
  of cheddar cheese, an egg, plus a few crackers (no butter)
  white coffee, no sugar

- **DINNER**
  grilled beef rib-steak
  carrots, beans, cauliflower and 1 potato
  white coffee, no sugar

- **LATE SNACK**
  a handful of peanuts

Total energy: 1400 kilocalories (6000 kilojoules)
Fat: 75 grams
Carbohydrate: 105 grams
Fibre: 20 grams

Looking at an analysis of this day we can see that:

1. **It is low in carbohydrate.**
   **Only 30 per cent of the total energy is supplied by
   carbohydrate. It is widely recommended that at least
   50 per cent of our daily energy should come from
   carbohydrate.**

To improve this diet it is essential to add some carbohydrate.

- Include a bowl of cereal and a piece of fruit with breakfast.
- Change the crackers at lunch to 2 slices of bread.
- Substitute the peanuts with a low-fat yoghurt as the late night snack.
- Add a cob of corn to the evening vegetables.
- Try some canned peaches for dessert.

2. **It is high in fat.**
   46 per cent of the total energy is provided by fat.
   It is widely recommended that less than 30 per cent of energy should come from fat.

To improve this diet, take away some fat.

- Halve the amount of butter used on toast.
- Use a low-fat cheese slice **or** ham **or** egg for lunch, not cheese and egg.
- Cut down the meat serving — select a small piece of fillet instead.
- Give up the peanuts! Substitute low-fat yoghurt instead, or canned fruit, or low-fat ice cream with fruit salad.

To work out the percentage of energy supplied by carbohydrate, the grams of carbohydrate are multiplied by 4 (the number of kilocalories supplied per gram of carbohydrate) and then divided by the total number of kilocalories

Thus: $(105 \times 4 \times 100)/1500 = 28$ per cent

■■■ WHAT ABOUT THE DIFFERENT TYPES OF CARBOHYDRATE?

Traditionally, carbohydrate has been classified in terms of its chemical structure. We now know from scientific research and clinical trials with real people that the whole concept of simple and complex carbohydrates does not tell us anything about how they will actually behave in the body. Until recently, it was widely believed that complex carbohydrates, or starches such as rice and potato, were slowly digested and absorbed and therefore caused only a small rise in blood sugar level. Simple sugars, on the other hand, were assumed to be digested and absorbed quickly, producing a large and rapid increase in blood sugar. These assumptions were largely incorrect.

Forget about the words

simple and complex carbohydrate.

Think in terms of

low G.I. and high G.I. factor.

■■■■ THE CARBOHYDRATE/G.I. FACTOR LINK

Newer studies are revealing that the physiological responses to food (how food acts in the body) are far more complex than was previously appreciated. What is true is that different carbohydrate-containing foods do have different effects on blood sugar levels.

Only in recent years have scientists begun to study the actual blood sugar responses to hundreds of different foods on real people, healthy people and people with diabetes. They gave them real foods — not solutions of sugars and starches in water. They measured the blood sugar levels at frequent intervals, for as long as two to three hours after the meal. Then to compare foods according to their true physiological effect on blood sugar levels, they came up with the term 'glycaemic index'.

The glycaemic index (or G.I. factor as we have called it) is a ranking of foods from 0 to 100 that tells us whether a food will raise blood sugar levels dramatically, moderately, or just a little.

This research has turned some widely held beliefs upside down.

The first surprise was that many starchy foods (bread, potatoes and many types of rice) are digested and absorbed very quickly, not slowly as had always been assumed.

Secondly, they found that moderate amounts of most sugary foods (confectionery, ice cream etc.) did not produce dramatic rises in blood sugar as had always been thought. The truth was that foods containing sugar actually showed quite low-to-moderate blood sugar responses, lower than foods like bread.

So, it is time to forget the old distinctions that were made between starchy foods and sugary foods or simple versus complex carbohydrate. These distinctions are based on chemical analysis of the food, which does not totally reflect the effects of these foods on the body. The G.I. factor takes us nearer to a full understanding of how the body responds to carbohydrate foods.

The G.I. factor

is a ranking of foods

based on their overall effects

on blood sugar levels.

The next chapter tells you all about the G.I. factor.

BLOOD SUGAR OR BLOOD GLUCOSE?

Blood sugar and blood glucose mean the same thing, although the latter is technically more correct. However, we use the term blood sugar in this book because it is more widely understood.

CHAPTER 3

ALL ABOUT
THE G.I. FACTOR

THE KEY IS THE RATE OF DIGESTION

WHY THE G.I. FACTOR IS SO IMPORTANT

CAN THE G.I. FACTOR BE APPLIED TO REAL MEALS?

WHAT GIVES ONE FOOD A HIGH G.I. FACTOR AND
ANOTHER FOOD A LOW ONE?

THE EFFECT OF FAT AND PROTEIN
ON THE G.I. FACTOR

THE EFFECT OF SUGAR ON THE G.I. FACTOR

THE EFFECT OF FIBRE ON THE G.I. FACTOR

THE EFFECT OF ANTI-NUTRIENTS ON THE G.I. FACTOR

•

The glycaemic index concept (the G.I. factor) was first developed in 1981 by Dr David Jenkins, a professor of nutrition at the University of Toronto, Canada, to help determine which foods were best for people with diabetes. At that time, the diet for people with diabetes was based on a system of carbohydrate exchanges or portions, which was complicated and not very logical. The carbohydrate exchange system assumed that all starchy foods produce the same effect on blood sugar levels even though some earlier studies had already proven this was not correct. Jenkins was one of the first researchers to question this assumption and investigate how real foods really behave in the bodies of real people.

Jenkins' approach attracted a great deal of attention because it was so logical and systematic. He and his colleagues had tested a large number of common foods. Some of their results were surprising. Ice cream, for example, despite its sugar content, had much less effect on blood sugar than ordinary bread. Over the next fifteen years medical researchers and scientists around the world, including the authors of this book, tested the effect of many foods on blood sugar levels and developed a new concept of classifying carbohydrates based on the glycaemic index (G.I. factor) of a food.

For some years the glycaemic index was a very controversial area. There were avid proponents and opponents of this new approach to classifying carbohydrate. The two sides almost came to blows at conferences aimed at reaching a consensus.

Initially, there was some criticism which was justified. In the early days, there was no evidence that G.I. factors for single foods could be applied to mixed meals or that the approach brought long-term benefits. There were no studies of its reproducibility or the consistency of G.I. factors from one country to another. Many of the early studies used healthy volunteers and there was no evidence that the results could be applied to people with diabetes. But now that the evidence is in and we know the G.I. factors of more than 600 foods, all the early doubts have been put to rest. To date, clinical studies in the United Kingdom, France, Italy, Australia and Canada all have proven without doubt the value of the glycaemic index. Notably, the USA remains one of the last bastions of opposition. This may have more to do with academic politics than science!

The glycaemic index (or G.I. factor) of foods is simply a ranking of foods based on their immediate effect on blood sugar levels. To make a fair comparison, all foods are compared with a reference food such as pure glucose and are tested in equivalent carbohydrate amounts.

Today we know the G.I. factors of hundreds of different food items that have been tested following the standardised method. The table on pages 24 to 25 gives the G.I. factors of a range of common foods, including many tested by the University of Sydney. The table of G.I. factors in Part III gives the G.I. factors of more than 250 foods.

■■■■ THE KEY IS THE RATE OF DIGESTION

Carbohydrate foods that break down quickly during digestion have the highest G.I. factors. The blood sugar response is fast and high. In other words the glucose (or sugar) in the bloodstream increases rapidly. Conversely, carbohydrates which break down slowly, releasing glucose gradually into the bloodstream, have low G.I. factors. An analogy might be the popular fable of the tortoise and the hare. The hare, just like high G.I. foods, speeds away full steam ahead but loses the race to the tortoise with his slow and steady pace. Similarly, the slow and steady low G.I. foods produce a smooth blood sugar curve without wild fluctuations.

For most people most of the time, the foods with low G.I. factors have advantages over those with high G.I. values. But there are some athletes who can benefit from the use of high G.I. foods during and after competition. This is covered in Chapter 6.

The substance which produces the greatest rise in blood sugar levels is pure glucose itself. All other foods have less effect when fed in equal amounts of carbohydrate. The G.I. factor of pure glucose is set at 100 and every other food is ranked on a scale from 0 to 100 according to its actual effect on blood sugar levels.

The G.I. factor of a food cannot be predicted from its composition or the G.I. factor of related foods. To test the G.I. factor, you need real people and real foods. We describe how the G.I. factor of a food is measured in the following box. There is no easy, inexpensive substitute test. Standardised methods are always followed so that results from one group of people can be directly compared with those of another group.

....

HOW SCIENTISTS MEASURE THE G.I. FACTOR

I. An amount of food containing 50 grams of carbohydrate is given to a volunteer to eat. For example, to test boiled potatoes, the volunteer would be given 250 grams of potatoes which supplies 50 grams of carbohydrate (we work this out from food composition tables) — 50 grams of carbohydrate is equivalent to 3 tablespoons of pure glucose powder.

2. Over the next two hours (or three hours if the volunteer has diabetes), we take a sample of their blood every 15 minutes during the first hour and thereafter every 30 minutes. The blood sugar level of these blood samples is measured in the laboratory and recorded.

3. The blood sugar level is plotted on a graph and the area under the curve is calculated using a computer program (Figure 1).

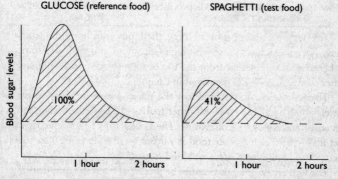

GLUCOSE (reference food)   SPAGHETTI (test food)

FIGURE 1. Measuring the G.I. factor of a food. The effect of a food on blood sugar levels is calculated using the area under the curve (hatched area). The area under the curve after consumption of the test food is compared with the same area after the reference food (usually 50 grams of pure glucose or a 50 gram carbohydrate portion of white bread).

4. The volunteer's response to potato (or whatever food is being tested) is compared with his or her blood sugar response to 50 grams of pure glucose (the reference food).

5. The reference food is tested on two or three separate occasions and an average value is calculated. This is done to reduce the effect of day-to-day variation in blood sugar responses.

THE GLYCAEMIC INDEX OF SOME POPULAR FOODS

(Glucose = 100)

KEY

*Foods containing relatively high amounts of fat

G.I. RANGES: The figures form a continuum, but in general:

LOW G.I. FOODS .... below 55
INTERMEDIATE G.I. FOODS ....between 55 and 70
HIGH G.I. FOODS .... more than 70

BREAKFAST CEREALS

Kellogg's All-Bran™	42
Kellogg's Coco Pops™	77
Kellogg's Corn Flakes™	84
Mini Wheats™	58
Muesli – toasted*	43
untoasted	56
Porridge	42
Kellogg's Rice Krispies™	82
Kellogg's Special K™	54
Kellogg's Sultana Bran™	52
Kellogg's Sustain™	68

GRAINS / PASTAS

Buckwheat	54
Bulgur (burghul)	48
Rice – Basmati	58
brown	76
brown quick cooking	80
white	87
Noodles – instant	46
Pasta – egg fettuccine	32
ravioli (meat)	39
spaghetti	41
vermicelli	35
Taco shells	68

BREAD

Bagel	72
Croissant*	67
Crumpet	69
Fruit loaf (white)	47
Heavy grain bread	46
Pitta bread	57
Rye bread – kernel e.g.	
pumpernickel	41
Flour e.g. blackbread	76
White bread	70
Wholemeal bread	69

CRACKERS / CRISPBREAD

Puffed crispbread	81
Ryvita	69
Water biscuit	78

SWEET BISCUITS

Arrowroot	63
Morning coffee	79
Oatmeal	55
Shortbread (commercial)*	64
Wheatmeal	62

CAKES ETC

Apple muffin*	44
Banana cake*	47
Sponge cake	46
Waffles	76

VEGETABLES

Beetroot	64
Carrots	49
Parsnip	97
Peas (green)	48
Potato – baked	85
new	62
French fries	75
Pumpkin	75
Swede	72
Sweet corn	55
Sweet potato	54
Yam	51

LEGUMES

Baked beans	48
Broad beans	79
Butter beans	31
Chick peas	33
Haricot beans	38
Kidney beans	27
Lentils	28
Soya beans	18

FRUIT

Apple	38
Apricot (dried)	31
Banana	55
Cantaloupe melon	65
Cherries	22
Grapefruit	25
Grapes	46
Kiwifruit	52
Mango	55
Orange	44
Pawpaw (papaya)	58
Peach – canned in juice	30
fresh	42
Pear	38
Pineapple	66
Plum	39
Raisins	64
Sultanas	56
Watermelon	72

DAIRY FOODS

Milk –	whole	27
	skimmed	32
	chocolate flavoured	34
	custard (made with powder)	43
Ice cream		61
	low-fat	50
Yoghurt flav, low-fat		33

BEVERAGES

Apple juice	40
Fanta™	68
Lucozade™	95
Orange juice	46
Squash (diluted)	66

SNACK AND CONVENIENCE FOODS

Corn chips*	72
Fish fingers	38
Peanuts*	14
Popcorn	55
Potato crisps*	54
Sausages*	28
Soup – lentil	44
pea	66
tomato	38

CONFECTIONERY

Chocolate*	49
Jelly beans	80
Mars Bar*	68
Muesli bar*	61

SUGARS

Honey	58
Fructose	23
Glucose	100
Lactose	46
Maltose	105
Sucrose	65

In total, eight to twelve people need to be tested and the G.I. factor of the food is the average value of the group. We know this average figure is reproducible and that a different group of volunteers will produce a very similar result. Results obtained in a group of people with diabetes are comparable to those without diabetes.

The important point to note is that all foods are tested in equivalent carbohydrate amounts. For example, 100 grams of bread (about 3½ slices of sandwich bread) is tested because this contains 50 grams of carbohydrate. Likewise, 60 grams of jelly beans (containing 50 grams of carbohydrate) is compared with the reference food. We know how much carbohydrate is in a food by consulting food composition tables, manufacturer's data or measuring it ourselves in the laboratory.

GLUCOSE OR WHITE BREAD?

Some scientists have decided to use a 50 gram carbohydrate portion of white bread as the reference food because it is more physiological — typical of what we actually eat. On this scale, where the G.I. factor of white bread is set as 100, some foods will have a G.I. value over 100 because their effect on blood sugar levels is higher than that of bread.

The use of two standards has caused some confusion but it is possible to convert from one to the other using the factor 1.4 (100/70 — white bread has a G.I. value of 70 when glucose is the reference food).

To avoid confusion throughout this book, we refer to all foods according to a standard where glucose equals 100. The G.I. factor table in Part III gives values for both standards.

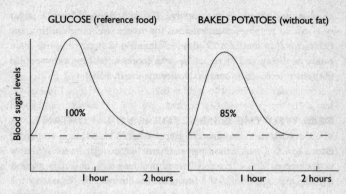

FIGURE 2. The effect of pure glucose (50 grams) and baked potatoes (50 gram carbohydrate portion) on blood sugar levels.

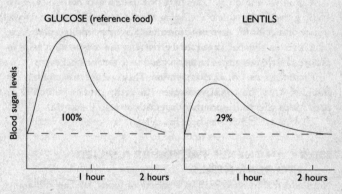

FIGURE 3. The effect of pure glucose (50 grams) and lentils (50 gram carbohydrate portion) on blood sugar levels.

The higher the G.I. factor, the higher the blood sugar levels after consumption of the food. Foods with a high G.I. will have both a high peak and will maintain a higher blood sugar level for longer.

Rice Krispies™ (G.I. factor equals 82) and baked potatoes (G.I. factor equals 85) have very high G.I. factors, meaning their effect on blood sugar levels is almost as high as that of an equal amount of pure glucose (yes, you read it correctly). Figure 2 shows the blood sugar response to potatoes compared with pure glucose. Foods with a low G.I. factor (like lentils at 29) show a flatter blood sugar response when eaten, as shown in Figure 3. The peak blood sugar level is lower and the return to baseline levels is slower than with a high G.I. food.

▋▋▋▋ WHY THE G.I. FACTOR IS SO IMPORTANT

The **slow** digestion and **gradual** rise and fall in blood sugar responses after a low G.I. factor food helps control blood sugar levels in people with diabetes. This effect may benefit healthy people as well because it reduces the secretion of the hormone insulin over the course of the day. (This is discussed in greater detail on page 59 and in chapter 7.) Slower digestion helps to delay hunger pangs and promote weight loss in overweight people.

A food with a low G.I. factor, eaten one to two hours before an event, gives the tri-athlete a winning edge by providing a slow-release source of fuel for the exercising muscles, thereby extending endurance. In contrast, a high G.I. factor food given after the competition helps to restore muscle fuel stores faster, in good time for the next event.

These facts are not an exaggeration. They are not just preliminary findings. They are confirmed results of many studies published in prestigious scientific journals by scientists around the world.

▋▋▋▋ CAN THE G.I. FACTOR BE APPLIED TO REAL MEALS?

Normally, real meals consist of a variety of foods. We can still apply the G.I. factor to these real meals even though the G.I. values are originally derived from testing single foods in isolation. Scientists have found that it is possible to predict the blood sugar rise for a meal based on several foods with different G.I. factors. The total carbohydrate content of the meal and the contribution of each food to the total carbohydrate must be known. Data like this can be found in food composition tables.

For example, say you have a breakfast based on orange juice, Weetabix™ with milk and a slice of toast with a thin scrape of butter.

In the following table, you can see how the G.I. factor of the total meal has been calculated. This may look complicated. In practice, people don't need to make these sorts of calculations at all. But dietitians and nutrition researchers sometimes have to. Many studies have shown a very close relationship between the predicted blood sugar response (as based on published G.I. factors of the relative effects of different foods and meals) and the actual observed blood sugar response.

HOW WE CALCULATE THE OVERALL G.I. FACTOR OF A MEAL BASED ON SEVERAL FOODS WITH DIFFERENT G.I. VALUES

Mixed meal	Carbohydrate (g)	% total carbohydrate	G.I. factor	Contribution to meal G.I.
Orange juice 150 ml (¼ pt)	12.5	23	46	23% x 46 = 11
Weetabix™ 30 g	21	39	69	39% x 69 = 27
Milk 150 ml (¼ pt)	7	13	27	13% x 27 = 4
1 slice of toast	13	24	70	24% x 70 = 17
Totals	53.5	100		**Meal G.I. = 59**

▆▆▆ WHAT GIVES ONE FOOD A HIGH G.I. FACTOR AND ANOTHER FOOD A LOW ONE?

Scientists have been studying what makes one food high and another low for more than fifteen years. There is a wealth of information that can easily confuse. We have summarised the results of their research in the following table which looks at the factors which influence the G.I. factor of a food.

The key message is that the physical state of the starch in the food is by far the most important factor influencing the G.I. value. That's why the advances in food processing over the past two hundred years have had such a profound effect on the overall G.I. factor of the food we eat.

FACTORS WHICH INFLUENCE THE G.I. OF A FOOD

Factor	Mechanism	Examples of foods where the effect is seen
Low degree of starch gelatinisation	The less gelatinised (swollen) the starch, the slower the rate of digestion.	Spaghetti, porridge, biscuits
Physical form of food	The fibrous coat around beans and seeds and intact plant cell walls act as a physical barrier, slowing down access of enzymes to the starch inside.	Pumpernickel bread, beans, lentils and foods cooked al dente (lightly)
High amylose to amylopectin ratio	The more amylose a food contains, the lower its rate of starch digestion.	Basmati rice
Fibre	Viscous, soluble fibres increase the viscosity of the intestinal contents and this slows down the interaction between the starch and enzymes. Finely milled wholemeal flours have fast rates of digestion and absorption.	Rolled oats, rye and barley breads, beans and lentils
Sugar	The digestion of sugar produces only half as many glucose molecules as the same amount of starch (the other half is fructose). The presence of sugar also restricts gelatinisation of the starch by binding water during food manufacture.	Some biscuits and some breakfast cereals
Fat	Fat slows down the rate of stomach emptying thereby slowing the digestion of starch.	Potato crisps have a lower G.I. factor than baked potatoes
Protein-starch and fat-starch interactions	Interactions of protein or fat with starch can slow digestion of the starch.	Legumes, pasta
Anti-nutrients	Some foods contain substances that inhibit digestion of starch e.g. phytates, tannins.	Soya beans, yams

The degree of starch gelatinisation The starch in raw food is stored in hard compact granules that make it difficult to digest. This is why potatoes will give you a pain in the stomach if you eat them raw. Most starchy foods need to be cooked for this reason. During cooking, water and heat expand the starch granules to different degrees, some granules actually bursting and freeing the individual starch molecules. This is what happens when you make a gravy by heating flour and water until the starch granules burst and the gravy thickens.

If most of the starch granules present have swollen and burst during cooking, the starch is said to be fully gelatinised. Figure 4 shows the difference between raw and cooked starch in potatoes.

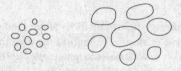

FIGURE 4. The difference between raw (compact granules) and cooked (swollen granules) starch in potatoes.

The swollen granules and free starch molecules are very easy to digest because the starch-digesting enzymes in the small intestine have a greater surface area to attack. The quick action of the enzymes results in a rapid and high blood sugar rise after consumption of the food (remember that starch is a string of glucose molecules). A food containing starch which is fully gelatinised will therefore have a very high G.I. factor.

In foods such as biscuits, the presence of sugar and fat and very little water makes starch gelatinisation more difficult, and only about half of the granules will be fully gelatinised. For this reason, biscuits tend to have intermediate G.I. factors.

Particle size Another factor that influences starch gelatinisation is the particle size of the food. Grinding or milling of cereals reduces the particle size and makes it easier for water to be absorbed and enzymes to attack. That is why cereal foods made from fine flours tend to have high G.I. factors. The larger the particle size, the lower the G.I. factor as shown in Figure 5.

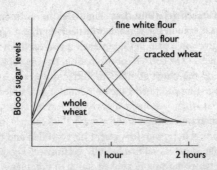

FIGURE 5. The larger the particle size, the lower the G.I. factor.

One of the most significant alterations to our food supply came with the introduction of steel roller mills in the mid-nineteenth century. Not only did they make it easier to remove the fibre from cereal grains, the particle size of the starch was smaller than ever before. Prior to the nineteenth century, stone grinding produced quite coarse flours that resulted in slower rates of digestion and absorption.

When starch is consumed in its natural packaging — whole intact grains that have been softened by soaking and cooking — the food will have a low G.I. factor. For example, cooked barley has a G.I. factor of only 25. Most cooked legumes have a G.I. factor between 30 and 40. Cooked whole wheat has a G.I. factor of 41.

The only whole (intact) grain food with a high G.I. factor is low amylose rice. It seems that these varieties of rice have starch which is very easily gelatinised during cooking and therefore easily broken down by digestive enzymes. This may help explain why we sometimes feel hungry not long after rice-based meals. However, some varieties of rice (Basmati, a long grain fragrant rice, and Doongara, a new Australian variety of rice) have intermediate G.I. factors because they have a higher amylose content (see below) than normal rice. Their G.I. factors are in the range of 54 to 64.

Amylose and amylopectin There are two sorts of starch in food — amylose and amylopectin — and researchers have discovered that the ratio of one to the other has a powerful effect on the G.I. factor of a food.

Amylose is a straight chain molecule, like a string of beads. These tend to line up in rows and form tight compact clumps that are harder to gelatinise and therefore digest (see Figure 6).

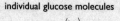

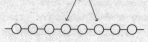

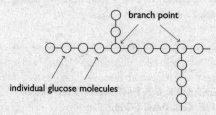

FIGURE 6. Amylose is a straight chain molecule which is harder to digest than amylopectin which has many branching points.

On the other hand, **amylopectin** is a string of glucose molecules with lots of branching points, such as you see in some types of seaweed. Amylopectin molecules are therefore larger and more open and the starch is easier to gelatinise and digest.

Thus foods that have little amylose and plenty of amylopectin in their starch have higher G.I. factors such as wheat flour. Foods with a higher ratio of amylose to amylopectin have lower G.I. factors including Basmati rice and all sorts of legumes.

WHY DOES PASTA HAVE A LOW G.I. FACTOR?

The starting point for making pasta is semolina or cracked wheat, not wheat flour. Durum wheat makes the best pasta because the grain is extremely hard and the wheat breaks cleanly into distinct small pieces. The large particle size of semolina means that starch gelatinisation is more difficult and thus enzyme attack is slowed down. That's why pasta of any shape and size has a fairly low G.I. factor (30 to 50). Cracked wheat and couscous used in Middle-Eastern cooking have intermediate G.I. factors.

■ THE EFFECT OF FAT AND PROTEIN ON THE G.I. FACTOR

High fat foods that have a low G.I. factor may appear in a falsely favourable light because increases in fat and protein tend to slow the rate of stomach emptying and therefore the rate at which foods are digested in the small intestine. High fat foods will therefore tend to have lower G.I. factors than their low-fat equivalents. For example, potato crisps have a lower G.I. factor (54) than potatoes baked without fat (85). Many sweet biscuits have a lower G.I. factor (55 to 65) than bread (70). But this is not a consistent finding. New boiled potatoes have a lower G.I. factor (62) than French fries (75), despite the latter's fat content.

Remember, however, we need to eat a low-fat diet, not a high fat one. So, high fat foods of any sort, whether low or high in their G.I. factor, should only be eaten in limited amounts.

■ THE EFFECT OF SUGAR ON THE G.I. FACTOR

Table sugar or refined sugar (sucrose) has a G.I. factor of only 65. This is because it is a disaccharide (double sugar) composed of one glucose molecule coupled to one fructose molecule. Fructose is absorbed and taken directly to the liver where much of it is slowly converted to glucose. So, the blood sugar response to pure fructose is very small (G.I. factor of 23). Thus when we consume sucrose, in effect we have consumed only half as much glucose. This explains why the blood sugar response to 50 grams of sucrose is approximately half that of 50 grams of pure gelatinised starch (where the molecules are all glucose).

Many foods containing large amounts of refined sugar have G.I. factors close to 60. This is lower than that of ordinary soft bread with a G.I. factor averaging around 70. Kellogg's Coco Pops™ which contains 39 per cent sugar has a G.I. factor of 77, lower than that of Rice Krispies™ (82) which contains little sugar.

So, contrary to popular opinion, most foods containing simple sugars do not raise blood sugar values any more than that of most complex starchy foods like bread. The same is true of honey (G.I. factor of 58). Some types of honey have a much higher G.I. factor (87) than refined sugar (65), possibly because they are a mixture of honey and glucose syrup.

Sugars that naturally occur in food include lactose, sucrose, glucose and fructose in variable proportions, depending on the food. The overall blood sugar response to a food is very hard to predict on theoretical grounds because gastric emptying is slowed by increasing concentration of the sugars, whatever their structure.

Some fruits for example have a low G.I. factor (cherries have a G.I. factor of only 22) while others are relatively high (watermelon has a factor of 72). It seems the higher the acidity and osmotic strength (number of molecules per ml) of the fruit, the lower the G.I. factor. Thus it is not possible to lump all fruits together and say that they will have a low G.I. factor because they are high in fibre. They are not all equal. See the tables in Part III to compare fruits.

Many foods containing sugars are a mixture of refined and naturally occurring sugars. The overall effect on the blood sugar response is too hard to predict. This is why we need to test the G.I. value of sugary foods before we make generalisations about their G.I. factor.

▰▰▰ THE EFFECT OF FIBRE
ON THE G.I. FACTOR

The effect of fibre on the G.I. factor of a food depends on the type of fibre. Finely ground cereal fibre, such as in wholemeal bread, has no effect whatsoever on the rate of starch digestion and subsequent blood sugar response. Similarly, any cereal product made with wholemeal flour will have a G.I. factor similar to that of its white counterpart. Breakfast cereals made with wholemeal flours will also tend to have high G.I. factors unless there are other influencing factors. Puffed wheat (80) and Weetabix™ (75) which are made from whole wheat grains have high G.I. factors.

If the fibre is still intact it can act as a physical barrier to digestion and then the G.I. factor will tend to be lower. This is one of the reasons why legumes have exceptionally low G.I. factors (30 to 40). It is also one of the reasons why whole (intact) grains usually have low G.I. factors, although most rice is an exception. Many varieties of rice, whether brown or white, have G.I. factors over 80.

Viscous fibre Viscous fibre thickens the viscosity or thickness of the mixture in the digestive tract. This slows the passage of food and restricts the movement of enzymes, thereby slowing digestion. The end result is a lower blood sugar response. Legumes contain high levels of viscous fibre, as do oats and psyllium (a seed which is a major ingredient in some breakfast cereals sold in the USA and Australia, and laxatives). These foods all have low G.I. factors.

▰▰▰ THE EFFECT OF ANTI-NUTRIENTS
ON THE G.I. FACTOR

Nature is not always benign. In unprocessed, natural foods there are plenty of substances that would be considered poisons if they were present in high enough concentrations. Substances which have potentially harmful effects on nutritional status are called anti-nutrients. Legumes, for example, contain enzyme inhibitors that can cause sickness if the food is not thoroughly cooked first to destroy them. Other anti-nutrients survive the cooking process and remain active in the body. These include phytates and tannins, compounds that bind minerals and may interfere with mineral absorption. Phytates and tannins occur in whole grains, brans, vegetables and legumes. The actual hazard depends on the amounts eaten. They can slow the rate of digestion of carbohydrate in the gastrointestinal tract and are another of the many reasons why legumes have lower G.I. factors than most foods.

CHAPTER 4

THE G.I. FACTOR AND YOU

YOUR QUESTIONS ANSWERED

●

Everybody can benefit from adopting the G.I. factor approach to eating. It is the way nature intended us to eat. She packaged all the nutrients we needed in a slow-release form. Since the Industrial Revolution, however, we have taken nature's carbohydrates and manufactured them into fast-release or instant food as part of our never-ending quest for a more palatable, more eye-catching and less perishable food supply. Unfortunately, the effect of all those instant foods is catching up on us in the form of diseases of affluence such as obesity and diabetes.

There is, however, no need to turn our backs on progress or go back to the days of the horse and cart. We have sufficient knowledge of food and nutrition to let the pendulum swing back just enough to suit our needs. But we need the facts. We need the answers to our questions. In this section we set out the facts in order to answer some of the most frequently asked questions about carbohydrates, diet and the G.I. factor to dispel any lingering doubts.

Is it better to eat complex carbohydrate like starches instead of simple sugars?

There are really no big distinctions between sugars and starches in either nutritional terms or in the G.I. sense (see page 34). Some sugars such as fructose or fruit sugar have a low G.I. factor. Others, such as glucose, have a high G.I. factor. The most common sugar in our diet, ordinary table sugar (sucrose), has an intermediate G.I. factor.

Starches can fall into both the high and low G.I. categories too, depending on the type of starch and what treatment it has received during cooking and processing. Most modern starchy foods, like bread, potatoes and breakfast cereals, contain high G.I. carbohydrate. What our research has shown is that you don't have to eliminate sugar completely from your diet. However, it is important to remember that sugar alone won't keep the engine running smoothly, so don't overdo it. Studies have shown that diets containing moderate amounts of refined sugars are perfectly healthy (10 to 12 per cent of kilocalorie intake) and the sugar helps to make many of the other nutritious foods in the diet more palatable.

DID YOU KNOW?

Did you know that fat and sugar tend to show a reciprocal or seesaw relationship in the diet? Studies over the past decade have found that diets high in sugar are no less nutritious than low sugar diets. This is because restricting sugar is frequently followed by higher fat consumption, and most fatty foods are poor sources of nutrients. In some cases, high sugar diets have been found to have higher micronutrient content, especially of calcium and riboflavin. This is because sugar is often used to sweeten some very nutritious foods, such as yoghurts, breakfast cereals and milk. A low sugar (and high fat) diet has more proven disadvantages than a high sugar (and low-fat) diet.

Are naturally occurring sugars in fruit better for us than refined sugars?

Naturally occurring sugars are those found in foods like fruit, vegetables and milk. Refined sugars are concentrated sources of sugar

such as table sugar, honey or molasses. The rate of digestion and
absorption of naturally occurring sugars is not different, on average,
from that of refined sugars. There is wide variation within both
food groups, depending on the food (see the figure below). For
example, the G.I. factor of fruits varies from 22 for cherries to 72
for watermelon. Similarly, among the foods containing refined
sugars, some have a low G.I. factor and some have a high G.I. factor.
The G.I. factor of sweetened yoghurt is only 33, while a Mars Bar™ has
a G.I. factor of 68 (almost the same as bread).

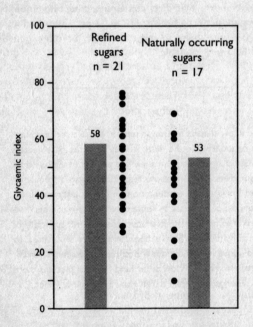

FIGURE 7. The figure shows the G.I. factors of foods containing either refined
sugars or naturally occurring sugars (fruit, fruit juice etc.). The bars show the
average value for each group. 'n' is the number of foods tested in each group.

Some nutritionists argue that naturally occurring sugars are better
because they contain minerals and vitamins not found in refined

sugar. However, new studies which have analysed high sugar and low sugar diets have clearly shown that they contain similar amounts of micronutrients. People who eat lots of refined sugars, tend to eat lots of food. Hence they eat more vitamins and minerals too.

Is honey better than sugar?

No, there is no benefit to substituting honey for sugar, unless you like the extra flavour that honey adds to a food. Both foods are concentrated sources of carbohydrate. Honey's G.I. factor appears to be similar to that of refined sugar (about 60), unless the honey is glucose enriched (which increases the G.I. factor). Honey was a major source of sweetness long before refined sugar became available at the beginning of the nineteenth century. In fact, historical research suggests that in some parts of the world we ate similar quantities of honey as we now do refined sugar. There are negligible quantities of other nutrients in honey. Honey is basically a mixture of glucose and fructose. These two single sugars are bound together as a disaccharide (double sugar) in refined sugar. The end result of digestion in the small intestine is similar for both honey and sugar.

Does sugar cause diabetes?

No. There is absolute consensus that sugar does not cause diabetes. Type 1 diabetes (insulin-dependent diabetes) is an autoimmune health problem triggered by unknown environmental factors such as viruses. Type 2 diabetes (non-insulin dependent diabetes) is strongly inherited but lifestyle factors such as lack of exercise and overweight increase the risk of developing it. Because the dietary treatment of diabetes in the past involved strict avoidance of sugar, many people wrongly believed that sugar was in some way implicated as a cause of the disease.

Are rice and pasta equal as carbohydrates?

In the general sense that they are both high carbohydrate, low-fat foods with valuable amounts of micronutrients, they are equal. Pasta has a higher protein content than rice but most people eat more than enough protein anyway. Pasta and rice are not equal in terms of the G.I. factors. The G.I. factor of all types of pasta is low, usually between 40 and 50. Rice, however, can have a high G.I. (80 to 90) or a low G.I. (50 to 55) depending on the variety and, in particular, its amylose content (see pages 32 and 33). In Britain and Ireland, as in Australia, there are many types of rice available and it is not always possible to identify the variety on the label. Long grain white rice has a high G.I. and Basmati rice has a lower G.I. The tables in Part III of this book (see pages 216 to 223) provide the G.I. factors of many types of rice. Brown rice and parboiled (converted) rice have a similar G.I. value to their white counterpart.

There is a lot of variation between people in terms of blood sugar responses to foods. Some people show very high responses, others low. The published G.I. factor reflects only the average response. How can the G.I. factor predict how any one individual will respond?

The way in which the G.I. factor of a food is determined helps to reduce the variation between people's responses. It allows for individual differences in glucose tolerance. Research has shown that the G.I. factor predicts the ranking of blood glucose responses of any one individual to a range of foods. For example, three foods with high, low and intermediate G.I. factors will have the same ranking in a person who tends to show high responses and another person who tends to show low responses. This is illustrated in the figure below.

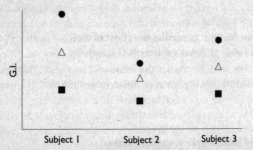

FIGURE 8. Three foods with high (●), intermediate (△) and low (■) G.I. factors will follow the same ranking in different individuals.

Why are there different G.I. values for the same food in different publications?

In some instances, there is a difference between two results but it is small and not statistically or biologically important. For example, G.I. factors of 70 and 80 for white bread are not considered very different. The difference is within the error of the methodology. A difference of 20 units, say 60 and 80, is considered important in a clinical sense and is usually statistically significant as well.

There may also be differences due to variations in the food itself. Rice is a good example of this. Genetically determined differences in the amylose content of rice means that different varieties of rice have very different G.I. factors. Basmati rice has a low G.I. factor and long grain white rice has a high G.I. factor. In the early days of G.I. research, the variety of rice was not specified.

Again, the same food processed in different ways can produce very different G.I. factors. Breads containing a lot of intact whole grains will have a lower G.I. factor than normal soft white sandwich bread. Packaged breakfast cereals, on the other hand, are processed in similar ways all over the world and their G.I. factors are very similar in Canada, Australia, Britain and elsewhere.

A third reason is the use of two reference foods, bread or glucose. However, it is easy to convert from one scale to the other using the factor 1.4 (equals 100/70). For example, if the G.I. factor of a food is 80 when bread is the reference food, its G.I. factor, on a scale where glucose equals 100, is 80 divided by 1.4 (equals 57).

Is the G.I. factor able to predict the effect of a mixed meal containing foods with very different G.I. factors?

Yes, the G.I. factor can predict the relative effects of different mixed meals containing foods with very different G.I. factors. Over fifteen studies have looked at the G.I. factors of mixed meals. Twelve of these studies showed an excellent correlation between what was expected and what was actually found. You can predict the G.I. of a mixed meal by making a few simple calculations (see page 29).

The other three studies which did not show the expected correlation came from a particular group of researchers who were not using standardised methodology for working out the G.I. factor from the area under the curve. In addition, their meals were high in fat instead of carbohydrate, and this tends to reduce the impact of any one carbohydrate food.

Has the G.I. factor been tested in long-term studies?

At least twelve studies to date have looked at the G.I. factor in the diet in relation to long-term diabetes control. Some of these studies have been five weeks long, others, including ours, up to three months. All but one showed a clear benefit in improving blood sugar levels. People with high blood lipids (cholesterol, triglycerides) showed improvements in this area as well.

The insulin response is important and the G.I. factor does not tell us anything about this. Is there a correlation?

In general, studies have found an excellent correlation between the G.I. factor of a food and its insulin response. Sometimes the insulin response is higher or lower than expected. The presence of more protein will increase the insulin response proportionately. A large amount of fat may slow glycaemic response but not the insulin response. But we should be avoiding large amounts of fat.

Why do different groups around the world come up with different values for the same food?

For the most part, we see very reproducible G.I. factors for the same foods from standardised tests around the world. Apples and oranges, for example, have been tested a great deal and give similar G.I. factors. Packaged foods like cornflakes also give very consistent values.

Rice is one food which is very variable because its amylose content varies from variety to variety.

Oats and porridge vary, too. To date we are not sure of the reasons for this.

Potatoes vary with the variety and method of cooking.

I'm confused about the G.I. of rice. Some people say it has a high G.I. factor, others say it is low.

Rices usually have a high G.I. factor because their amylose content is low. On page 32 we described how amylose is a form of starch which is more difficult to digest and results in lower G.I. factors. Basmati, a fragrant long grain rice from India, is high in amylose and has a low G.I. factor. You can guess at the G.I. factor of rice by its appearance after cooking. If it is sticky and individual grains clump together, the rice is likely to have a high G.I. factor. On the other hand, if the rice is dry and the grains separate, it is likely to have a relatively low G.I. factor.

A high fat food may have a low G.I. factor. Doesn't this give a falsely favourable impression of that food for people with diabetes?

Yes it does. The G.I. factor of potato crisps or French fries is lower than baked potatoes. The G.I. of corn chips is lower than sweet corn. It is important not to base your food choices on the G.I. factor alone. It is essential to look at the fat content of foods as well. Low-fat eating is best for everyone, especially people with diabetes.

What effect does fibre have on the G.I. value?

Dietary fibre is not one chemical constituent like fat and protein. It is composed of many different sorts of molecules. Fibre can be divided into soluble and insoluble types.

Soluble fibre tends to be viscous (thick and jelly-like) and will slow down digestion for this reason. Foods with more soluble fibre, like oats and legumes, therefore have low G.I. factors.

Insoluble fibre is not viscous and doesn't slow digestion. Wholemeal bread and white bread have similar G.I. factors. Brown pasta and brown rice have similar values to their white counterparts. Sometimes insoluble fibre acts as a physical barrier which prevents the enzymes from attacking the starch. Whole (intact) grains of wheat, rye and barley have lower G.I. factors than cracked grains.

Are G.I. factors tested on healthy people valid for use in people with diabetes?

Yes, there are several studies which show a good correlation between values for the same foods obtained in healthy people and people with diabetes. This is no surprise because the degree of glucose intolerance is allowed for in the calculation of G.I. factors.

Do low G.I. foods need to be eaten at every meal in order for people to see a benefit?

No, because the effect of a low G.I. food carries over to the next meal, reducing its glycaemic impact. This applies even when the low G.I. meal is eaten for dinner. Its effect carries over to breakfast the following morning. But, it is sensible to try to eat at least two low G.I. factor meals each day.

Bread has a G.I. of around 70 and lentils of around 29. Can I eat twice as much of the low G.I. food as the high G.I. food?

Yes, your blood sugar levels should be approximately the same after two servings of lentils or pasta compared with one serving of bread or potatoes. But, you will have eaten twice as many kilocalories (kilojoules). In practice, you will find that it is very difficult to eat a double serving of foods like lentils and pasta because they are very satiating and fill you up. If you can eat twice as much, it may be a good thing, because you are unlikely to have room for high-fat and less nutritious foods!

Which type of carbohydrate should athletes be eating?

This depends on the type of sport being pursued. If an athlete is undertaking prolonged, strenuous events over two hours at maximum oxygen consumption (over 2 hours at >65% VO2 max) he or she may benefit from eating low G.I. foods one to two hours beforehand. High G.I. foods, however, are needed after the event to replenish glycogen stores. During everyday training sessions, both high and low G.I. foods are suitable. This is dealt with in more detail in Chapter 6. It may be helpful for athletes to consult a sports dietitian.

One study gave carrots a G.I. factor of 95. Does this mean that a person with diabetes shouldn't eat carrots?

Even with a G.I. factor of 95, a normal serving of carrots would contribute only a small amount to the rise in blood sugar. Carrots and other foods like tomatoes and salad vegetables that contain only a small amount of carbohydrate should be seen as 'free' foods for people with diabetes.

The quantity of carrots that gives the 50 grams of carbohydrate portion (as required in standardised G.I. factor testing) is enormous because it contains only about 7 per cent carbohydrate. In fact, about 700 grams of carrots were tested. This is much greater than the amount you would normally eat (about 100 grams).

If foods containing refined sugar have an intermediate G.I. factor, does this mean that people with diabetes can eat as much sugar as they want?

Research has clearly shown that the G.I. factor of refined sugar is the same in people that have diabetes and people that don't. Moderate consumption of sugar does not compromise blood sugar control. In fact, excluding sugar from the diet has important psychological consequences. Sugar is not just empty kilocalories, but a source of pleasure and reward and it helps to limit the intake of fatty foods and high G.I. carbohydrate foods. Our advice is to spread your sugar allowance over a variety of nutrient rich foods that become more palatable with the addition of sugar.

Bread and potatoes have high G.I. factors (70 to 80). Does this mean a person with diabetes should avoid bread and potatoes?

Potatoes and bread can play a major role in a high carbohydrate and low-fat diet, even if a secondary goal is to reduce the overall G.I. factor. Only about half the carbohydrate has to be exchanged from high G.I. to low G.I. to achieve measurable improvements in diabetes. So, there is still room for bread and potatoes. Of course, some types of bread and potatoes have a lower G.I. factor than others and these should be preferred if the goal is to lower the G.I. as much as possible.

In the overall management of diabetes, the most important message is that the diet should be low in fat and high in carbohydrate. This will help people not only to lose weight, but to keep it off and improve their overall blood glucose and lipid control.

There are so few low G.I. foods that anyone wanting to follow a low G.I. diet would have to narrow the range of foods that he or she eats. Isn't this a bad thing?

It is a myth that you have to narrow the range of foods you eat on a low G.I. diet. In fact, some people have told us the opposite. They have found that the advent of the G.I. factor has expanded the range of foods they can eat because foods containing sugar are not unduly restricted.

The rumour that all low G.I. foods are high in fibre and not very palatable also needs dispelling. It is true that legumes and All-Bran may not be everyone's favourite foods, but pasta, oats, fruit and many favourite Mediterranean recipes using cracked wheat and lentils etc. are low G.I. and delicious. To dispel such myths finally, we have included many mouth-watering recipes using legumes and lentils in Part II.

Does the area under the curve give a true picture of the blood sugar responses? Why not use just the peak value?

The area under the curve is thought to reflect the sum total of the glycaemic response, not just the one time point given by the peak. Statisticians recommend use of the area under the curve. There is a very close relationship between the area under the curve and the peak response. That is, if one is high, the other is high and vice versa.

What about resistant starch? What effect does it have on the G.I. factor of a food?

Resistant starch is the starch which completely resists digestion in the small intestine. It cannot contribute to the glycaemic effect of the food because it is not absorbed. Resistant starch should not be included in the 50 gram carbohydrate helping which is the standard for G.I. testing because all of this 50 grams should be available carbohydrate, that is available for absorption in the small intestine.

Resistant starch is not viscous like some forms of soluble fibre that delay absorption in the small intestine and flatten the blood glucose curve. Hence the mere presence of resistant starch in the food will not affect the G.I. factor of a food. Bananas and potato salad both have relatively high amounts of resistant starch but the G.I. factors of these two foods are very different. Potatoes have a high G.I. factor and bananas an intermediate one. The difficulty that arises in testing is determining the true available carbohydrate content of food which is high in resistant starch. If the amount of resistant starch is underestimated, it will produce a falsely low G.I. factor.

Does the G.I. factor predict the glycaemic effect of a normal serving of food?

Yes, studies have shown that even though the G.I. factor has been determined on the basis of a 50 gram carbohydrate portion, it can be used to predict the effect of a normal serving size with a meal. This is why the long-term studies of real people with diabetes eating real low G.I. meals have been successful.

CHAPTER 5

THE G.I. FACTOR AND WEIGHT REDUCTION

WHY IS BEING OVERWEIGHT A PROBLEM ANYWAY?

WHY DO PEOPLE BECOME OVERWEIGHT?

THE NEED FOR EXERCISE

WHAT FOODS DO CAUSE PEOPLE
TO BECOME OVERWEIGHT?

HOW CAN THE G.I. FACTOR HELP?

YOU CAN CHECK YOUR DIET

KEEPING THE QUANTITY,
CUTTING BACK ON KILOCALORIES

3 TIPS FOR PEOPLE TRYING TO LOSE WEIGHT

PLANNING LOW G.I. MEALS

●

If you are overweight (or consider yourself overweight) chances are that you have looked at countless books, brochures and magazines offering a solution to losing weight. New diets or miracle weight loss solutions seem to appear weekly. They are clearly good for selling magazines, but for the majority of people who are overweight the 'diets' don't work (if they did, there wouldn't be so many!).

At best (while you stick to it), a 'diet' will reduce your energy or kilocalorie intake. At its worst, a 'diet' will change your body composition for the fatter. That is because many diets employ the technique of reducing your carbohydrate intake to bring about quick weight loss. The weight you lose, however, is mostly water (that was trapped or held with stored carbohydrate) and eventually muscle (as it is broken down to produce glucose). Once you return to your former way of eating, you regain a little bit more fat. With each desperate repetition of a diet you lose more muscle. Over years, the resultant change in body composition to less muscle and more fat makes it increasingly difficult to lose weight.

Take it as read, that the real aim in losing weight is losing body fat. And perhaps it would be better described as 'releasing' body fat. After all, to lose something suggests that we hope to find it again some day!

This chapter is not prescribing yet another 'diet' for you to try. This chapter will give you some important facts about food and how your body uses it. Not all foods are equal. When it comes to what we eat and losing weight, it is not necessarily a matter of reducing how much you eat. Research has shown that **the type of food you give your body determines what it is going to burn and what it is going to store as body fat**. It has also revealed that certain foods are more satisfying to the appetite than others.

This is where the G.I. factor plays a leading role. Low G.I. foods have two very special advantages for people wanting to lose weight:

■ they fill you up and keep you satisfied for longer,
■ they help you burn more of your body fat and less of your body muscle.

Eating to lose weight with low G.I. foods is easier because you don't have to go hungry and what you end up with is true fat release.

■■■■ WHY IS BEING OVERWEIGHT A PROBLEM ANYWAY?

If you are overweight you are at increased risk of a range of health problems. Among these are heart disease, diabetes, high blood pressure, gout, gallstones, snoring and sleep apnoea, and arthritis. Along with this list of physical side effects of being overweight, there are an equal number of emotional and psychological problems.

The proportion of overweight people in our society is increasing, despite the expanding weight-loss industry and an ever increasing range of 'diet' or 'lite' foods. It is clear that the answer to preventing people from becoming overweight is not a simple one. Nor is losing weight easy to do. The G.I. factor changes all that. It tells you which foods satisfy hunger for longer and are the least likely to make you fat. When you use the G.I. factor as the basis for your food choices:

■ there is no need to restrict your food intake excessively,
■ there is no need to count kilocalories obsessionally,
■ there is no need to starve yourself.

Learning with which foods your body works best is what using the G.I. factor is all about.

It is worthwhile taking control over aspects of your lifestyle that have an impact on your weight. You may not create a new body from your efforts, but you will feel better about the body you've got. Eating and exercising for your best performance is the aim of the game.

■■■■ WHY DO PEOPLE BECOME OVERWEIGHT?

Is it genetic?
Is it hormonal?
Is it our environment?
Is it a psychological problem?
Or is it due to an abnormal metabolism?

Consider the energy balance paradox that exists in our bodies. For most of us, even without much conscious effort, our bodies maintain a constant weight. This is despite huge variations in how much we eat. For a proportion of people who are overweight this apparent balancing of energy intake and output seems lost or inoperative. So, despite every fad diet, every exercise programme, even operations and medications, body weight can steadily increase over the years, regardless of all apparent efforts to control it.

It has always been said that our weight is a result of how much we take in and how much we burn up. So, if we take in too much (overeat) and don't burn up enough (don't exercise) we are likely to put on weight.

The question is: how much, of what, is too much?

The answer is not a simple one: not all foods that we eat are equal and no two bodies are the same.

People are overweight for many different reasons. Some people believe they only 'have to look at food', others put on weight from 'just walking past the pâtisserie', others blame themselves because they eat too much. It is clear that a combination of social, genetic, dietary, metabolic, psychological (**and emotional**) factors combine to influence our weight.

'It must be in my genes' Before we talk more about food, let's look at the role genetics plays in weight control. There are many overweight people who tell us resignedly that:

- 'well, my mother's/father's the same',
- 'I've always been overweight',
- 'it must be in my genes'.

Research shows us that this comment has much truth behind it. A child born to overweight parents is much more likely to be overweight than one whose parents were not overweight. It may sound like an excuse, but there is a lot of evidence to back the idea that our body weight and shape is at least partially determined by our genes.

Much of our knowledge in this area comes from studies in twins. Identical twins tend to be similar in body weight even if they are raised apart. Even twins adopted as infants show the body-fat profile of their true parents rather than that of their adoptive parents. These findings suggest that our genes are a stronger determinant of weight than our environment (which includes the food we eat).

It seems that information stored in our genes governs our tendency to store kilocalories as either fat or as lean muscle tissue. Overfeeding a large group of identical twins confirmed that within each pair, weight gain was similar; however, the amount of weight gained between sets of identical twins varied greatly. From this, researchers concluded that our genes control the way our bodies respond to overeating. Some sets of twins gained a lot of weight while others gained only a little, even though all were overconsuming an equivalent amount of kilocalories.

MEASURING THE FUEL WE NEED

Kilocalories are a measure of the fuel we need. Our bodies need a certain number of kilocalories every day to work, just as a car needs so many litres of petrol to run for a day. Food and drink are our source of kilocalories. If we eat and drink too much we may store the extra kilocalories as body fat. If we consume fewer kilocalories than we need, our bodies will break down its stores of fat to make up for the shortfall.

Metabolism Our genetic make-up also underlies our **metabolism** (basically how many kilocalories we burn per minute). Bodies, like cars, differ in this regard. A V-8 consumes more fuel to run than a small 4-cylinder car. A bigger body, generally, requires more kilocalories than a smaller one. Everybody has a **resting metabolic rate**. This is a measure of the amount of kilocalories our bodies use when we are at rest. When a car is stationary, the engine idles — using just enough fuel to keep the motor running. When we are asleep, our engine keeps running (for example, our heart keeps beating) and we use a minimum number of kilocalories. This is our resting metabolic rate. Our resting metabolic rate is the amount of kilocalories we burn without any exercise. When we start exercising, or even just moving around, the number of kilocalories, or the amount of fuel we use, increases. However, the largest amount (around 70 per cent) of the kilocalories used in a 24-hour period are those used to maintain our basic body functioning.

Since our resting metabolic rate is where most of the kilocalories we eat are used, it is a significant determinant of our body weight. The lower your resting energy expenditure the greater your risk of gaining weight and vice versa. We all know someone who appears to 'eat like a horse' but is positively thin! Almost in awe we comment on their 'fast metabolism', and we may not be far off the mark!

All this isn't to say that if your parents were overweight you should resign yourself to being overweight. But it may help you understand why you have to watch your weight while other people seemingly don't have to watch theirs.

So, if you were born with a tendency to be overweight, why does it matter what you eat? The answer is that foods (or more correctly, nutrients) are not equal in their effect on body weight. In particular the way the body responds to dietary fat makes matters worse. **If you are overweight it is likely that the amount of fat you burn is small, relative to the amount of fat you store**. Consequently, the more fat you eat, the more fat you store. Although this may sound logical, the 'eat-more, store-more' mechanism does not exist for all nutrients.

DID YOU KNOW?

The body loves to store fat. It is a way of protecting us in case of famine. In the midst of plenty we are building up our fat stores.

Amongst all four major sources of kilocalories in food (protein, fat, carbohydrate and alcohol), fat is unique. When we increase our intake of protein, alcohol or carbohydrate the body's response is to **burn** more of that particular energy source. Sensibly, the body matches the supply of fuel with the type of fuel burned. One of the fundamental differences between fat and carbohydrate is that fat tends to be stored whereas carbohydrate has a tendency to be burned. It is worth noting at this point that if your carbohydrate intake is low, it may reduce the amount of kilocalories you burn each day by 5 to 10 per cent.

Whilst you may not have been born owning the best set of genes, you can still influence your weight by the lifestyle choices you make. The message is simply this: if you believe that you are at risk of being overweight, you should think seriously about minimising fat and eating more carbohydrate.

THE NEED FOR EXERCISE

A 'fast metabolism' is not necessarily a matter of luck. Exercise, or any physical activity, speeds up our metabolic rate. By increasing our kilocalorie expenditure, exercise helps to balance our sometimes excessive kilocalorie intake from food.

Exercise also makes our muscles better at using fat as a source of fuel. By improving the way insulin works, exercise increases the amount of fat we burn. A low G.I. diet has the same effect. Low G.I. foods reduce the amount of insulin we need which makes fat easier to burn and harder to store. Since body fat is what you want to get rid of when you lose weight, exercise in combination with a low G.I. diet makes a lot of sense!

WHY EXERCISE KEEPS YOU MOVING

The effect of exercise doesn't stop when you stop moving. People who exercise have higher metabolic rates and their bodies burn more kilocalories per minute even when they are asleep!

WHAT FOODS DO CAUSE PEOPLE TO BECOME OVERWEIGHT?

It was widely (and wrongly) believed for many years that sugar and starchy foods like potato, rice and pasta were the cause of obesity. Twenty years ago, every diet for weight loss advocated restriction of these carbohydrate-rich foods. One of the reasons for this carbohydrate restriction stemmed from the 'instant results' of low carbohydrate diets. If your diet is very low in carbohydrate, you will lose weight. The problem is that what you primarily lose is fluid, and not fat. What's more a low carbohydrate diet depletes the glycogen stores in the muscles making exercise difficult and tiring.

Sugar has been blamed as a cause of people becoming overweight primarily because it is often found in high fat foods, where it serves to make the fat more palatable and tempting. Chocolate, which contains almost one-third of its weight in the form of fat, would be inedible if it didn't taste sweet.

Current thinking is that there is little evidence to condemn sugar or starchy foods as the cause of people becoming overweight. Overweight people show a preference for fat-containing foods rather than a preference for foods high in sugar. In a survey performed at the University of Michigan where obese men and women listed their favourite foods, men listed mainly meats (protein-fat sources) and women listed mainly cakes, biscuits, doughnuts (combinations of carbohydrate-fat sources). Other studies have found that obese people habitually consume a higher fat diet than people who have a healthy weight. So, it appears that a higher intake of fatty food is strongly related to the development of obesity — not carbohydrate-rich foods.

COUNTING THE KILOCALORIES IN OUR NUTRIENTS

All foods contain kilocalories. Often the kilocalorie content of a food is considered a measure of how fattening it is. Of all the nutrients in food that we consume, carbohydrate yields the fewest kilocalories per gram, similar to protein.

carbohydrate	4 kilocalories per gram
protein	4 kilocalories per gram
alcohol	7 kilocalories per gram
fat	9 kilocalories per gram

Whether you are going to gain weight from eating a particular food really depends on how much that food adds to your total kilocalorie intake in relation to how much you burn up. To lose weight you need to eat fewer kilocalories and burn more kilocalories. **If your total kilocalorie balance does not change — there will be no change in your weight**. People who consume a high fat diet automatically eat a high kilocalorie diet because there are more kilocalories per gram in fatty foods. This is why eating low-fat foods makes weight loss much easier.

■ HOW CAN THE G.I. FACTOR HELP?

One of the hardest parts of trying to lose weight can be feeling hungry all the time, but this gnawing feeling is not necessary when you are losing weight. **Carbohydrates are natural appetite suppressants**. And of all carbohydrate foods, those with a low G.I. factor are the most filling and prevent hunger pangs for longer.

In the past, it was believed that protein, fat and carbohydrate foods, taken in equal quantities, satisfy our appetite equally. We now know from recent research that the satiating (making us feel full) capacity of these three nutrients is not equal.

Fatty foods, in particular, have only a weak effect on satisfying appetite relative to the number of kilocalories they provide. This has been demonstrated clearly in experimental situations where people are asked to eat until their appetite is satisfied. They over-consume kilocalories if the foods they are offered are high in fat. When high carbohydrate and low-fat foods are offered, they consume fewer kilocalories, eating to appetite. So, carbohydrate foods are the best for satisfying our appetite without over-satisfying our kilocalorie requirement.

In studies conducted at the University of Sydney, people were given a range of individual foods that contained equal numbers of kilocalories, then the satiety (feeling of fullness and satisfaction after eating) responses were compared. The researchers found that the most filling foods were foods high in carbohydrate that contained fewer kilocalories per gram. This included potatoes, porridge, apples, oranges and pasta. **Eating more of these foods satisfies appetite without providing excess kilocalories**. On the other hand, high fat foods that provide a lot of kilocalories per gram, like croissants, chocolate and peanuts, were the least satisfying. These foods help us store more fat and are less filling to eat. **Many people notice that eating extra carbohydrate at a meal tends to be compensated by eating less food at the next meal**.

When we eat more carbohydrate, the body responds by increasing its production of glycogen. Glycogen is stored as glucose, the critical fuel for our brain and muscles. The size of these stores is limited, however, and they must be continuously refilled by carbohydrate from the diet. Good glycogen stores ensure a well-fuelled body and make it easier to exercise. Even when we are not exercising, the body will use carbohydrate in preference to other fuel sources, attempting to match the source of kilocalories to the type of kilocalories used.

Because fat is less satisfying to our appetite, it is easy to over-consume fatty kilocalories. That is why reducing the dietary fat intake is a far more effective means of achieving weight control while satisfying the appetite than restricting carbohydrate intake. By eating a high carbohydrate diet you will automatically be lowering your fat intake, and by choosing that carbohydrate from low G.I. foods, you make it even more satisfying.

What's more, even when the kilocalorie intake is the same, people eating low G.I. foods may **lose more weight** than those eating high G.I. foods. In a South African study, the investigators divided overweight volunteers into two groups: one group ate high G.I. foods and the other, low G.I. foods. The amount of kilocalories, fat, protein, carbohydrate and fibre in the diet was the same for both groups. Only the G.I. factor of the diets was different. The low G.I. group included foods like lentils, pasta, porridge and corn in their diet and excluded high G.I. foods like potato and white bread. After 12 weeks, the volunteers in the group eating low G.I. foods had lost, on average, 9 kilograms (20 pounds) — 2 kilograms (4½ pounds) more than people in the group eating the diet of high G.I. foods.

How did the low G.I. diet work? The most significant finding was the different effects of the two diets on the level of insulin in the blood. Low G.I. foods resulted in lower levels of insulin circulating in the bloodstream. Insulin is a hormone that is not only involved in regulating blood sugar levels, it also plays a key part in when and how we store fat. High levels of insulin often exist in obese people, in those with high blood fat levels (either cholesterol or triglyceride) and those with heart disease. This study suggested that the low insulin responses associated with low G.I. foods helped the body to burn more fat.

If you are still fearful of gaining weight from eating more pasta, bread and potatoes, consider this: the body actually has to use up kilocalories to convert the carbohydrate we eat into body fat. The cost is 23 per cent of the available kilocalories — that is, nearly one-quarter of the kilocalories of the carbohydrate are used up just storing it. Naturally, the body is not keen on wasting energy this way. In fact, the body converts carbohydrate to fat only under very unusual situations like forced overfeeding. The human body prefers the easy option. It is far more willing to add to our fat stores with the fat that we eat. Conversion of fat in food to body fat is an extremely efficient process and body fat stores are virtually limitless. No matter how excessive the amount of fat we eat, the body will always find space to store it.

WHICH FOODS ARE MOST FATTENING?

For the same amount of kilocalories, you can eat far more carbohydrate food than fatty food. To prove the point, let's compare two everyday foods which are almost pure in the nutrition sense. Three teaspoons of sugar (almost pure carbohydrate) has the same number of kilocalories as 1 teaspoon of oil (almost pure fat). This means that you can eat three times the volume of sugar as you could oil!

Here are some examples of how you can eat **more carbohydrate food** than fatty food for about the same number of kilocalories:

- A small grilled T-bone steak (about the size of a slice of bread) has the same kilocalories as 3 medium potatoes.
- 3 slices of bread, thickly buttered, are equivalent to 6 slices of bread with no butter.
- 3 chocolate cream biscuits have more kilocalories than a carton (400 ml/14 fl oz) of low-fat chocolate milk.
- Eating 1 piece of crumbed, fried chicken at lunch substitutes for the kilocalories of 6 slices of bread (without butter).
- For every serving of fried rice you eat you could eat 2 servings of boiled rice.
- And if you're feeling extra hungry next time you stop for a coffee, consider that one slice of chocolate fudge cake has the kilocalories of 4 slices of lightly buttered raisin toast!

In every case the highest fat foods have the highest kilocalorie count. Because carbohydrate has about half the kilocalories of fat, it is safer to eat more carbohydrate-rich food. What's more, the body will store fat and burn carbohydrate so the kilocalories contribute more to your 'spread' when they come from fat.

You can eat quantity — just consider the quality!

▰▰▰ YOU CAN CHECK YOUR DIET

HOW MUCH CARBOHYDRATE DID YOU EAT YESTERDAY?

1. Recall the amounts of carbohydrate foods that you ate yesterday. Remember to include all those little snacks as well as the main meals!

2. Using the serving size guide below estimate the number of servings you had in the whole day. For example, if you had a banana, 2 slices of bread and a medium potato, this counts as 4 servings of carbohydrate.

Carbohydrate food	One serving is	How many did you eat?
Fruit	a handful or 1 medium piece	
Juice	about 250 ml (9 fl oz)	
Dried fruit	around 1–2 tablespoons	
Bread	1 slice	
English muffin, bread roll, bagel	½ a roll, muffin or bagel	
Crackers, crispbread	2 large pieces or 4–6 small crackers	
Rice cakes	2 rice cakes	
Muffin, biscuits	½ a muffin or 2–3 biscuits	
Health bar/sports bar	approximately ½ average bar	
Breakfast cereal	1 bowl or 2 biscuits	
Porridge	1 tablespoon raw oats	
Rice	1 heaped tablespoon cooked rice	
Pasta, noodles	1 heaped tablespoon cooked noodles	
Pancakes	about ½ a large pancake	
Burghul, couscous	1 heaped tablespoon, cooked	

Potato, sweet potato	1 medium potato, about 100 g (3½ oz)
Sweet corn	1 small cob or 1 heaped tablespoon kernels
Lentils	2 tablespoons, cooked
Baked beans, other beans	1 heaped tablespoon, cooked
Total	

Rate yourself:

Less than 4 servings a day	=	Poor.
Between 4 and 8 servings a day	=	Fair, but you need to eat a lot more.
Between 9 and 12 servings a day	=	Satisfactory, could do better.
Between 13 and 16 servings a day	=	Great.
Over 16 servings a day	=	You're a whiz!

IS YOUR DIET TOO HIGH IN FAT?

Use this fat counter to tally up how much fat your diet contains.

Circle all the foods that you could eat in a day, look at the serving size listed and multiply the grams of fat up or down to match your serving size. For example, with milk, if you estimate you might consume 500 ml (18 fl oz) full cream milk in a day, this supplies you with 20 grams of fat.

Food	Fat content (grams)	How much did you eat?
Dairy Foods		
Milk, 250 ml (9 fl oz)		
full cream	10	
semi-skimmed	4	
skimmed	0	
Yoghurt, 200 g (7 oz)		
full-fat	10	
low-fat	0	
Ice cream, 2 scoops, 100 ml (3½ fl oz)		
full-fat	10	
low-fat	3	

Cheese

regular, block cheese, 30 g (1 oz) slice	10
reduced fat block cheese,	
30 g (1 oz) slice	7.5
low-fat slices (per slice)	2.5
cottage, 2 tablespoons	4

Cream/sour cream, 1 tablespoon

full-fat	8
fat-reduced	4

Fats and Oils

Butter/margarine, 1 teaspoon	4
Oil, any type, 1 tablespoon (20 ml)	20
Cooking spray, per spray	1
Mayonnaise, 1 tablespoon	7
Salad dressing, 1 tablespoon	5

Meat

Beef

steak, average, 1 small, lean only	10
minced beef, 160 g (6 oz),	
cooked, drained	15
sausage, 1 thick, grilled, 80 g (3 oz)	14
topside roast, 2 slices, lean only	
80 g (3 oz)	4

Lamb

chump chop, grilled, lean only, 2	9
leg, roast meat, lean only, 2 slices,	
80 g (3 oz)	5
loin chop, grilled, lean only, 2	5

Pork

bacon, 1 rasher, grilled	9
ham, 1 slice, leg, lean	2
butterfly steak, lean only	5
leg, roast meat, 3 slices, lean only	4
loin chop, lean only	4

Chicken

breast, skinless	4
drumstick, skinless	7
thigh, skinless	7
½ barbecue chicken (including skin)	15

Fish

grilled fish, 1 average fillet	1.5
salmon, 50 g (2 oz)	5
fish fingers, 4, grilled	12
fish fillets, 2, crumbed, oven baked	
regular	20
light	10

Snack Foods

Potato crisps, 50 g (2 oz)	16
Corn chips, 50 g (2 oz)	14
Peanuts, 70 g (2½ oz)	32
French fries, average serving	20
Pizza, 2 slices, medium pizza	25
Pie/sausage roll	24

Total

How did you rate?

Less than 40 grams	=	Excellent.
		30 to 40 grams of fat per day is recommended for those trying to lose weight.
41 to 60 grams	=	Good.
		A fat intake in this range is recommended for most adult men and women.
61 to 80 grams	=	Acceptable.
		If you are very active, i.e. doing hard physical work (labouring) or athletic training. It is too much if you are trying to lose weight.
More than 80 grams	=	You're possibly eating too much fat, unless of course you are Superman or Superwoman!

▬▬▬ KEEPING THE QUANTITY, CUTTING BACK ON KILOCALORIES

If you are trying to reduce your kilocalorie intake there is still a **minimum** amount of certain foods that you should be eating each day. These are:

▩ Breads/cereals/and grain foods — 5 servings or more

1 serving means 1 bowl breakfast cereal (30 g/1 oz)
1 heaped tablespoon cooked pasta or rice
1 heaped tablespoon cooked grain such as barley or wheat
1 slice bread
½ bread roll or English-style muffin

▩ Vegetables — 4 servings

1 serving means 1 medium potato (about 150 g/5½ oz)
60 g (2 oz) cooked vegetables such as broccoli or carrot
2–3 leaves raw leafy vegetables, such as lettuce

▩ Fruit — 3 servings

1 serving means: 1 medium orange (200 g/7 oz)
1 medium apple (150 g/5½ oz)
½ punnet strawberries (100 g/3½ oz)

▩ Dairy foods — 2 servings

1 serving means: 300 ml (½ pt) milk
40 g (1½ oz) cheese
200 g (7 oz) low-fat yoghurt

▩ Meat and alternatives — 1 serving

1 serving means 60–80 g (2–3 oz) cooked lean beef, veal, lamb or pork
120 g (4 oz) lean chicken (raw weight, excluding bone)
150 g (5½ oz) fish (raw weight, excluding bone)
2 eggs
2 heaped tablespoons cooked lentils or dried peas or beans

■■■ 3 TIPS FOR PEOPLE TRYING TO LOSE WEIGHT

1. Eat regular meals — include snacks in between if you are hungry.

2. Try to include a low G.I. food at every meal.

3. Ensure that your meals contain mainly carbohydrate and vegetable foods and that the fat content is low.

■■■ PLANNING LOW G.I. MEALS

Breakfast
- Start with a bowl of low G.I. cereal served with skimmed or semi-skimmed milk or low-fat yoghurt.
- Try something like All-Bran™, rolled oats or Sultana Bran™.
- If you prefer muesli, keep to a small bowl of natural muesli — not toasted.
- Add a slice of toast made from a low G.I. bread (or 2 slices for a bigger person) with a dollop of jam, sliced banana, honey, yeast extract spread, marmalade, or light cream cheese with sliced apple. Keep butter or margarine to a minimum, or use none at all.
- If you like a hot breakfast, try baked beans, a boiled or poached egg, cooked tomatoes or mushrooms with your toast.

Lunch
- Try a sandwich or roll, leaving the butter off. If you can, choose a bread with lots of whole grains through it (not just sprinkled on top) for a low G.I. factor. Add plenty of salad fillings.
- For the filling choose from a thin slice of leg ham, pastrami, lean roast beef or chicken or turkey, or a slice of low-fat cheese, salmon or tuna (in brine), or an egg. An extra container of salad or vegetable soup will help to fill you up.

■ Finish your lunch with a piece of fruit, or fruit salad with a low-fat yoghurt, or a low-fat flavoured or plain milk.

Dinner

■ The basis of the dinner should be the carbohydrate and vegetables.

■ Eat as many vegetables as you can, using a small amount of meat, chicken or fish as a flavouring rather than the main ingredient.

■ Use lean meat like topside beef, veal, pork, trimmed lamb, chicken breast, fish fillets, turkey. Red meat is a valuable source of iron — just choose lean types. A piece of meat, chicken or fish that fits in the palm of your hand fulfils the daily protein requirements of an adult.

■ If you prefer not to eat meat, 2 heaped tablespoons cooked dried peas, beans, lentils or chick peas can provide protein and iron without any fat. At the same time they supply low G.I. carbohydrate and fibre.

■ Use meat replacements: these are generally based on high protein legumes like soya beans and nuts etc.

■ Boost your fruit intake and get into the habit of finishing your meal with fruit — fresh, stewed or baked. Or try a fruit ice, e.g. sorbet.

Snacks

■ It is important to include a couple of dairy food servings each day for your calcium needs. If you haven't used yoghurt or cheese in any meals, you may choose to make a low-fat milkshake. One or two scoops of low-fat ice cream or custard can also contribute to daily calcium intake.

■ If you like grainy breads, an extra slice makes a very good choice for a snack. Other snacks can include toasted English-style muffin halves, a crumpet with a smear of butter, bagels or fruit loaf.

■ Fruit is always a low kilocalorie option for snacks. You should aim to consume at least 3 servings a day. It may be helpful to prepare fruit in advance to make it accessible and easy to eat.

■ Low-fat crackers (like water biscuits) are a low kilocalorie snack if you want something dry and crunchy, although they may not be as sustaining as a grainy bread. Popcorn (home-prepared with a minimum of fat) is another good alternative.

■ Keep vegetables (like celery and carrot sticks, baby tomatoes, florets of blanched cauliflower or broccoli) ready prepared to snack on, too.

CHAPTER 6

THE G.I. FACTOR AND PEAK SPORTS PERFORMANCE

WHY IS THE G.I. FACTOR RELEVANT
TO SPORTING PERFORMANCE?

A HIGH CARBOHYDRATE DIET IS ESSENTIAL
FOR PEAK SPORTING PERFORMANCE

THE G.I. FACTOR REPRESENTS FINE-TUNING
OF THE HIGH CARBOHYDRATE DIET

THE CASE FOR LOW G.I. FOODS

THE CASE FOR HIGH G.I. FOODS

MISCONCEPTIONS ABOUT CARBOHYDRATES

THE PRE-EVENT MEAL

DURING AN EVENT

RECOVERY (AFTER THE EVENT)

HOW MUCH FOOD DO YOU NEED TO EAT
TO GET THIS MUCH CARBOHYDRATE?

THE TRAINING DIET AND
CARBOHYDRATE LOADING

HOW DO YOU CHOOSE A HIGH
CARBOHYDRATE DIET?

Australian scientists were the first in the world to apply the concept of the glycaemic index to sport and exercise. British and Canadian scientists 'invented' the G.I. approach to help classify carbohydrates but Australian researchers could see that what they were doing had important implications for sporting performance. The rest of the world is still catching up. Manipulating the G.I. of the diet can give you the winning edge — whether you are one of the elite or a weekend warrior.

███ WHY IS THE G.I. FACTOR RELEVANT TO SPORTING PERFORMANCE?

The G.I. factor ranks foods on the basis of the measured blood sugar response to a specific food. The rate at which glucose enters the bloodstream affects the insulin response to that food and ultimately affects the fuels available to the exercising muscles. There are times when low G.I. foods provide an advantage and times when high G.I. foods are better. For best performance, a serious athlete needs to learn about which foods have high and low G.I. factors and when to eat them.

High G.I. factor foods like potatoes will produce a rapid increase in glucose and insulin levels, something which is not desirable just before a race when glycogen stores should already be fully charged. Low G.I. foods, such as pasta, which are digested and absorbed much more slowly, are able to provide glucose to the working muscle towards the end of exercise when glycogen stores are running low. They can be likened to a continuous injection of glucose during the event. This can boost energy when fatigue begins to set in. After the event, high G.I. foods are best because they stimulate more insulin, the hormone responsible for putting glycogen back into the muscles.

Manipulating the G.I.

of your diet can give you

the winning edge!

■■■ A HIGH CARBOHYDRATE DIET IS ESSENTIAL FOR PEAK SPORTING PERFORMANCE

A high carbohydrate diet is a must for optimum sports performance because it produces the biggest stores of muscle glycogen. As we have previously described, the carbohydrate we eat is stored in the body in the form of glycogen in the muscles and liver. A small amount of carbohydrate (about 1 teaspoonful) circulates as glucose in the blood. When you are exercising at a high intensity, your muscles rely on glycogen and glucose for fuel. Although the body can use fat when exercising at lower intensities, fat cannot provide the fuel fast enough when you are working very hard. The bigger your stores of glycogen and glucose, the longer you can go before fatigue sets in.

Unlike the fat stores in the body which can release almost unlimited amounts of fatty acids, the carbohydrate stores are small. They are fully depleted after two or three hours of strenuous exercise. This drying up of carbohydrate stores is often called 'hitting the wall'. The blood glucose concentration begins to decline at this point. If exercise continues at the same rate, blood glucose may drop to levels which interfere with brain function and cause disorientation and unconsciousness. Some athletes refer to this as a 'hypo'.

All else being equal, the eventual winner is the person with the largest stores of muscle glycogen. Any good book on nutrition for sport will tell you how to maximise your muscle glycogen stores by ingesting a high carbohydrate training diet and by 'carbohydrate loading' in the days prior to the competition. In this chapter we provide instructions for increasing muscle glycogen. However, first we show you how you can extend your endurance even further with the G.I. factor.

■■■ THE G.I. FACTOR REPRESENTS FINE-TUNING OF THE HIGH CARBOHYDRATE DIET

The G.I. factor is now used to describe differences between carbohydrate foods, based on their rate of digestion and physiological effect on blood sugar levels. What relevance has this to athletes? During competition, many athletes can be seen supplementing their carbohydrate stores by consuming sugars in one form or another, sports drinks, bananas etc. These foods provide extra glucose for the exercising muscles when they need it most. In fact, research has proven beyond all doubt that carbohydrate consumption during strenuous exercise extends endurance for a lot longer than otherwise possible. But what about food before an event? Can what you eat before exercise extend endurance? The answer is yes!

▮▮▮▮ THE CASE FOR LOW G.I. FOODS

Imagine that it is possible to carry a reservoir or an extra store of carbohydrate to use when needed in the small intestine (not the stomach).

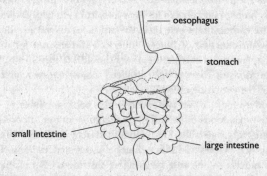

FIGURE 9. The gastrointestinal tract of the human body.

A meal containing carbohydrate must be eaten about two hours before strenuous exercise, such as a race, allowing time for the food to leave the stomach and reach the small intestine. You may experience nausea and stomach cramps if you eat too close to the race, e.g. less than an hour beforehand.

The problem is that by allowing a gap of about two hours, the carbohydrate in most foods would have been burnt as fuel well before the race begins. The small intestine would be empty and no longer acting as a reservoir of carbohydrate. There is one other possibility. What if you could package the carbohydrate in such a way as to make it be released more slowly from the small intestine during the event?

What is needed is a food that is so slowly digested that it remains in the small intestine for hours after consumption. Only some foods have their carbohydrate packaged in such a way as to make it slowly digested and absorbed and gradually released from the small intestine. In the same way that certain drugs have been formulated as **lente** (the Italian word for **slowly**) or 'slow-release' compounds so that the drug's action is evenly maintained throughout the day, it is possible to do this with the carbohydrate in food, too.

It shouldn't come as a surprise to learn that nature originally provided carbohydrate in a slow-release form or lente carbohydrate. Starch and sugars in raw, unprocessed foods are packaged in a cell matrix surrounded by fibre and only gradually broken down by the enzymes of the gastrointestinal tract. In the days of hunter-gatherers, when early humans literally ran for their lives from predatory animals, slow-release carbohydrate gave them the ultimate survival advantage. Before the introduction of horses, American Indians ran for miles rounding up bison and herding them over the cliffs to their death. The traditional foods of these people provided a slow-release source of glucose for the exercising muscle.

But modern foods, as we said earlier in this book, are different. We have made cereal foods more and more digestible in our attempts to make them more palatable. Most modern starchy foods like bread, cornflakes, rice crispies and other cereals are digested and absorbed extremely quickly — the true meaning of 'fast foods'! For example, ordinary soft white bread has a high G.I. factor of around 70 and many packaged breakfast cereals have G.I. factors between 80 and 90. These figures are nearly as high as pure glucose which has a G.I. factor of 100. What this means is that digestion of such starchy food is almost instantaneous and the blood sugar rise is consequently very rapid. Foods with a high G.I. factor do not provide the lente carbohydrate that represents the winning edge in a race.

Fortunately, there are still some foods in our diet that remain slowly digested and absorbed. These foods have a G.I. factor of less than 50. They include all kinds of pasta, barley, whole grains, porridge, All-Bran™ and some varieties of rice, and bread made with softened whole grains. They also include many foods made with lentils, chick peas, couscous and barley. The traditional Mediterranean diet was high in legumes, which have exceptionally low G.I. factors.

Low G.I. foods have been proven by Australian researchers to extend endurance when eaten alone one to two hours before prolonged strenuous exercise. When a pre-event meal of lentils (low G.I. factor) was compared with one of potatoes (high G.I. factor), cyclists were able to continue cycling at high intensity (65 per cent of their maximum) for 20 minutes longer after eating the lentil meal. Their blood sugar and insulin levels were significantly higher at the end of exercise, indicating that carbohydrate was still being absorbed from the small intestine even after 90 minutes of strenuous exercise. Figure 10 shows the blood sugar levels during exercise after consumption of low and high G.I. foods.

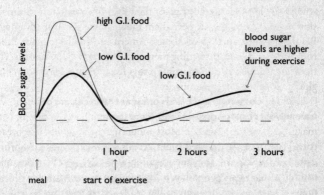

FIGURE 10. Comparison of the effect of low and high G.I. foods on blood sugar levels during prolonged strenuous exercise.

▬▬ THE CASE FOR HIGH G.I. FOODS

How do athletes in heavy training keep up the pace, day after day after day? Learning how to use your everyday food to aid your recovery has been the focus of recent research. The findings show that these are times when fast-release carbohydrate provides an advantage to an athlete. After hard exercise, carbohydrate stores in the muscles need to be replenished. This is done by consuming high carbohydrate foods as soon as possible after the race. Scientists at the Australian Institute of Sport in Canberra showed that high G.I. foods result in faster rates of glycogen synthesis compared to low G.I. foods (see Figure 11). This makes perfect sense because high G.I. foods are digested and absorbed much faster and stimulate more insulin, the hormone responsible for getting glucose into the muscle and storing it there in the form of glycogen.

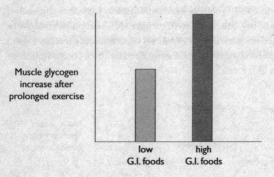

Muscle glycogen
increase after
prolonged exercise

           low   high
     G.I. foods   G.I. foods

FIGURE 11. Comparison of the effect of low and high G.I. foods on replenishment of muscle glycogen levels after exercise.

If you want to keep up the pace from one training session to another, day after day, you will benefit by learning to select high G.I. foods. The trouble is that many people, even coaches and sports medicine practitioners, have got it all wrong when it comes to selecting sources of fast-release carbohydrate. The information in this chapter gives you the most up-to-date information and the key to better performance and faster recovery. Go for it!

Forget about the words

simple and complex carbohydrate.

Think in terms of

low G.I. and high G.I. factor.

■■■ MISCONCEPTIONS ABOUT CARBOHYDRATES

In the past we were taught that simple carbohydrates (sugars) were digested and absorbed rapidly while complex carbohydrates (starches) were digested slowly. We assumed (completely incorrectly) that simple carbohydrates gave the most rapid rises in blood sugar while complex carbohydrates produced gradual rises. Unfortunately, these assumptions had no factual or scientific basis. They were based on structural considerations, smaller molecules, like sugars, being thought to be easier to digest than larger ones, like starches. Even though incorrect, the logical nature of these assumptions meant that they were rarely ever questioned.

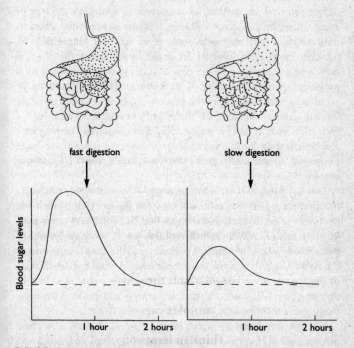

FIGURE 12. Slow and fast carbohydrate digestion and the consequent levels of sugar in the blood.

It was not until a highly respected British endocrinologist, Professor David Jenkins, published the first list of G.I. values that people began to listen. Now working in Canada, he and his colleagues showed that many foods containing starch gave blood sugar responses almost as high as an equivalent load of the simple sugar, glucose. Further research showed that many sugary foods had lower blood sugar rises than starchy foods. In other words, scientists and medical practitioners all over the world had it the wrong way round. Unfortunately, many still do.

▰▰▰ THE PRE-EVENT MEAL

Before you read any further, it's important to appreciate the type of event where the G.I. factor will help. It is one in which the athlete is undertaking a very strenuous form of exercise for longer than 90 minutes. Exercise physiologists define this by saying that the athlete is exercising at more than 65 per cent of their maximum capacity for a prolonged period. Examples of such events include a running or swimming marathon, a triathlon, non-stop tennis competition or football game (depending on the player's position). Some forms of recreation such as cross-country skiing and mountain climbing may also benefit from the G.I. approach. In some occupations that require prolonged strenuous activity for hours and hours, low G.I. foods may save lives.

Low G.I. foods are best before an event — approximately two hours before the big race. The meal will have left the stomach by then but continues to be digested in the small intestine for hours afterwards. The slow rate of carbohydrate digestion in low G.I. foods helps ensure that a steady stream of glucose is released into the bloodstream during the event. The extra glucose is available when needed towards the end of the exercise when muscle carbohydrate stores are running low. In this way, low G.I. foods increase endurance and prolong the time before exhaustion hits.

It's also important to select low G.I. foods that do not cause gastrointestinal discomfort such as stomach cramps and flatulence. Some low G.I. foods such as legumes are high in fibre or indigestible sugars. However, not all low G.I. foods are fibrous and high residue.

The high amylose rices (e.g. Basmati) and any form of white pasta are good examples of low G.I. foods that don't contain much fibre. Instant noodles have a low G.I., too. Athletes who are too nervous to eat a solid meal, may prefer a sustaining liquid supplement with a low G.I. (around 40, depending on the variety).

Helen O'Connor, a dietitian who works with many of Australia's Olympic athletes, teaches them how to manipulate the G.I. factor of their diet. Her book *The Taste of Fitness* is packed with low G.I. recipes. Craig Weller, a consultant sports dietitian in Sydney, recommends the following low G.I. foods before a race — baked beans on toast, rolled oats or pasta with tomato purée.

EVENTS WHERE THE G.I. FACTOR CAN GIVE YOU THE EDGE

running marathon

swimming marathon

triathlon

non-stop tennis competition

football game (depending on the player's position)

cross-country skiing

mountain climbing

prolonged strenuous aerobics
   and gym work-outs (longer than 90 minutes)

The food industry is keenly interested in the G.I. factor, too, and it won't be long before there are specially formulated low G.I. foods on the supermarket shelves specifically aimed at the serious sports person. The sports drinks that are enjoying much popularity at present have not been tested for their G.I. factor. Theoretically the mixture of sugars present would give a high G.I. of about 70. So they may not be an advantage before the event, but they are an invaluable aid during the event when blood sugar needs to be topped up, as well as after the event when glycogen stores need to be replenished.

THE PRE-EVENT MEAL

How much should I eat before the event?

About 1 gram of carbohydrate for each
kilogram (2 pounds) of body weight
(i.e. 50 grams of carbohydrate if you weigh 50 kilograms/8
stone, or 75 grams of carbohydrate if you weigh 75 kilo-
grams/12 stone)

How soon before?
1 to 2 hours before the event is a good starting point.

You should experiment to determine the timing
that works best for you.

The following tables show the serving sizes of low and intermediate G.I. foods containing 50 grams or 75 grams of carbohydrate.

You will not win if your pre-event meal is jiggling around in your stomach (this will affect the jogger more than the cyclist). So test the timing and amount of low G.I. food during your training sessions. Then you'll be ready for the big day. Don't try it out for the first time on the day of the competition!

**SERVING SIZES OF LOW G.I. FOODS
TO EAT 1 TO 2 HOURS
BEFORE THE EVENT**

Food	G.I.	Serving size = 50 grams carbohydrate	Serving size = 75 grams carbohydrate
Heavy grain breads eg. Pumpernickel	46	100 g (3½ oz) (3 slices)	150 g (5½ oz) (4 to 5 slices)
Spaghetti, cooked	37	200 g (7 oz)	300 g (10½ oz)
Porridge	42	600 g (1¼ lb)	900 g (2 lb)
Baked beans	48	450 g (medium can)	670 g (1½ medium cans)
Sustaining sports drink	approx 40	250 ml (9 fl oz)	400 ml (14 fl oz)
Fruit salad	approx 50	500 g (18 oz)	750 g (1½ lb)
Yoghurt	33	400 g (14 oz)	600 g (1¼ lb)
Apples	38	400 g (14 oz) (3 small medium)	600 g (1¼ lb) (4 medium)
Oranges	44	600 g (1¼ lb) (5 small)	900 g (2 lb) (7 small)
Dried apricots	31	105 g (3½ oz)	160 g (5½ oz)

Females weighing about 50 kilograms (8 stone) should aim to eat 50 grams of carbohydrate.

Males weighing about 75 kilograms (12 stone) should aim to eat 75 grams of carbohydrate.

TABLE OF INTERMEDIATE G.I. FOODS

Food	G.I.	Serving size = 50 grams carbohydrate	Serving size = 75 grams carbohydrate
Muesli	56	75 g (2½ oz) (+ 200 ml/7 fl oz milk)	110 g (4 oz) (+ 250 ml/9 fl oz milk)
Sultana Bran™	52	45 g (1½ oz) (+ 200 ml/7 fl oz milk)	75 g (2½ oz) (+ 250 ml/9 fl oz milk)
Rice (e.g. Basmati)	54–64	180 g (6 oz)	270 g (10 oz)
Honey	58	2½ tablespoons	4 tablespoons
Jam	59	3 tablespoons	6 tablespoons
Orange juice	46	600 ml (1 pt)	900 ml (1½ pt)

USING THE G.I. FACTOR ON THE DAY OF THE EVENT

Low G.I. · Breakfast
Large bowl of porridge with low-fat milk
Pasta with tomato-based sauce
Juice

Low G.I. · 1–2 hours pre-event
Dried apricots
Fruit salad
Fruit smoothie made with any low G.I.
  fruit and low-fat milk

High G.I. · During the event
(aim for 30 g carbohydrate and
  500ml/18 fl oz water per hour)
  e.g. at least 500 ml/18 fl oz sports
  drink
or 12 jelly beans + at least 500 ml/18 fl
  oz water
or honey sandwich + at least 500 ml/18
  fl oz water

**High G.I. · After the event
(within 30–60 minutes)**
1 litre (2 pt) sports drink
or Lucozade™
or 70 g (2½ oz) creamed rice
or 2 honey sandwiches
or bowl of rice crispies
  or cornflakes

High or Low G.I. · Dinner
270 g (10 oz) rice with meat or
  tuna topping (Fast food: eat double
  the rice but halve the normal serving of Chinese, Thai etc. main meal)
Vegetables
2 slices bread
350 g (12 oz) fruit salad and
  1 carton of yoghurt

▰▰▰ DURING AN EVENT

High G.I. foods should be used during events lasting longer than 90 minutes. This form of carbohydrate is rapidly released into the bloodstream and ensures that glucose is available for oxidation in the muscle cells. Liquid foods are usually tolerated better than solid foods while racing because they are emptied more quickly from the stomach. Sports drinks are ideal during the race because they replace water and electrolytes as well. The old standby of a banana strapped to the bike doesn't have much scientific basis. Its G.I. is only 60 and some of its carbohydrate is completely resistant to digestion (which could give you gas and a pain in the belly). If you feel hungry for something solid during a cycling race, try jelly beans (G.I. of 80) or a honey (preferably glucose enriched) sandwich (G.I. of 75).

Consume 30 to 60 grams carbohydrate

per hour during the event.

▰▰▰ RECOVERY (AFTER THE EVENT)

In some competitive sports, athletes compete on consecutive days and glycogen stores need to be at their maximum each time. Here it is important to restock the glycogen store in the muscles as fast as possible after the event. High G.I. foods are best in this situation. Sports scientists at the Australian Institute of Sport in Canberra have shown that high G.I. foods resulted in faster replenishment of glycogen into the fatigued muscles. Muscles are more sensitive to glucose in the bloodstream in the first hour after exercise, so a concerted effort should be made to get as many high G.I. foods in as soon as possible.

Suggested foods include most of the sports drinks on the market (which replace water and electrolyte losses too), or low amylose rice, breads and breakfast cereals with a high G.I. such as cornflakes and rice crispies. Potatoes cooked without fat are a good choice too, but their high satiating effect means it is hard to eat lots of them. Soft drinks have an intermediate G.I., so they won't be ideal but they won't do any harm either.

Which high G.I. foods are best after and between exercise bouts?

SERVING SIZES OF HIGH G.I. FOODS TO EAT BETWEEN AND DURING EVENTS

Food	G.I.	Serving size = 50 grams carbohydrate	Serving size = 75 grams carbohydrate
White or brown bread	70	100 g (3½ oz) (3 slices)	150 g (5½ oz) (4–5 slices)
Rice crispies	89	45 g (1½ oz) (+ 175 ml/6 fl oz milk)	65 g (2½ oz) (+ 300 ml/½ pt milk)
Corn Flakes (Kellogg's)	84	45 g (1½ oz) (+ 175 ml/6 fl oz milk)	65 g (2½ oz) (+ 300 ml/½ pt milk)
Scones	70	150 g (5½ oz) (2 large scones)	200 g (7 oz) (3 large scones)
Morning coffee biscuits	79	65 g (2¼ oz) (7 biscuits)	100 g (3½ oz) (11 biscuits)
Rice cakes	82	60 g (2 oz) (5 rice cakes)	90 g (3 oz) (8 rice cakes)
Puffed crispbread	81	65 g (2¼ oz) (13 crispbread)	100 g (3½ oz) (19 crispbread)
Water biscuits	78	70 g (2½ oz) (16 crackers)	110 g (4 oz) (24 crackers)
Muffins (English-style, toasted)	70	120 g (4½ oz) (2 muffins)	180 g (6 oz) (3 muffins)
Baked potato (without fat)	85	330 g (11 oz) (3 small–medium)	580 g (20 oz) (5 small)
Rice (not Basmati), cooked	83	180 g (6 oz)	270 g (9½ oz)
Jelly beans	80	55 g (2 oz) (25 jelly beans)	85 g (3 oz) (38 jelly beans)
Watermelon	72	1 kg (2 lb)	1.5 kg (3 lb)

Females weighing about 50 kilograms (8 stone) should aim to eat 50 grams of carbohydrate.

Males weighing about 75 kilograms (12 stone) should aim to eat 75 grams of carbohydrate.

RECOVERY FORMULA

Aim to ingest about 1 gram of carbohydrate per kilogram (2 pounds) of body weight each 2 hours after exercise. If you weigh between 50 and 75 kilograms (8 and 12 stone), you need 50 to 75 grams of carbohydrate for each 2 hours after exercise.

▄▄▄▄ HOW MUCH FOOD DO YOU NEED TO EAT TO GET THIS MUCH CARBOHYDRATE?

The table on page 84 gives the serving size of food and drinks containing 50 grams and 75 grams of carbohydrate. You need to choose a larger than normal serving. You may not feel like a meal of rice or pasta and this is the point where sports drinks and soft drinks on the market can help. Choose what you can tolerate and what is easy and practical for you to bring or buy. The main point is to make sure you eat and drink carbohydrate soon after the exercise session.

Sample menus for high G.I. post-event meals are listed on page 82.

TO MAXIMISE GLYCOGEN REPLENISHMENT AFTER THE COMPETITION

1. Ingest carbohydrate as soon as you can after the event and maintain a high carbohydrate intake for the next 24 hours.

2. Consume at least 10 grams of carbohydrate per kilogram (2 pounds) of body weight over the 24 hours following prolonged exercise.

3. Choose high G.I. foods in the replenishment phase.

4. Avoid alcohol (alcohol delays glycogen re-synthesis).

■■■■ THE TRAINING DIET AND CARBOHYDRATE LOADING

It's not just your pre-and post-event meals that influence your performance. Consuming a high carbohydrate diet every day will help you reach peak performance. The G.I. factor of the carbohydrate is not important here, only the amount of carbohydrate. It has been proven scientifically, unlike many other rumours involving dietary supplements, that eating lots of high carbohydrate foods will maximise muscle glycogen stores and thereby increase endurance.

The reason for this is that carbohydrate stores need to be replenished after each training session, not just after a race. If you train on a number of days per week, make sure you consume a high carbohydrate diet throughout the whole week.

Remember that alcohol interferes with glycogen re-synthesis and lowers blood glucose levels, sometimes to dangerous levels. Keep alcohol intake moderate — no more than one to three standard drinks per day and try to have two alcohol-free days a week. A standard drink is equivalent to one glass of wine (120 ml/4 fl oz), one 'half' of beer (285 ml) or one single measure of spirits (30 ml/1 fl oz).

Beer is not a good source of carbohydrate.

When athletes fail to consume adequate carbohydrate each day, muscle and liver glycogen stores may eventually became depleted. Dr Ted Costill at the University of Texas showed that the gradual and chronic depletion of stored glycogen may decrease endurance and exercise performance. Intense work-outs, often two to three times a day, draw heavily on the athlete's muscle glycogen stores. Athletes on a low carbohydrate diet will not perform at their best because muscle stores of fuel are low.

If the diet provides inadequate amounts of carbohydrate, the reduction in muscle glycogen will be critical. A heavily training athlete should consume about 500 to 800 grams of carbohydrate a day (about 60 per cent of total energy intake) to help prevent carbohydrate depletion. In practice, few athletes achieve this enormous figure. As a comparison, a typical man or woman eats only 240 grams of carbohydrate each day.

■ HOW DO YOU CHOOSE A
HIGH CARBOHYDRATE DIET?

The early chapters of this book provide all the practical tips you need for ensuring a high carbohydrate intake. In this chapter we give some extra pointers because very active people need to eat much larger amounts of carbohydrate than usual.

You may feel that you already know a lot about diet. But athletes, like everyone else, can have their facts wrong. Many foods that you believe are good sources of carbohydrate are even better sources of fat. For example, chocolate is 55 per cent carbohydrate but also 30 per cent fat. And fat won't help you win the race.

Dietary advice aimed at the general public needs to be modified for the serious sports person. Athletes have far greater energy needs, perhaps double that of the average office worker. Many high carbohydrate and low-fat foods which are recommended for the average person are too bulky and satiating for athletes. It is their bulk that makes it difficult to consume the required amount of food. For example, a 75 gram carbohydrate portion of potatoes is equivalent to 600 grams (1¼ lb) in weight of potatoes — about four normal servings. Most people can't eat that much at a time. On the other hand, white bread is easy to eat in large amounts. A 75 gram carbohydrate portion of white bread is only five slices. Other foods that you might have believed were not so good for you, like soft drinks, confectionery, honey, sugar, flavoured milk and ice cream, are actually very concentrated sources of carbohydrate that can be used to supplement your diet.

THE G.I. FACTOR AND DIABETES

WHAT IS DIABETES?

WHY DO PEOPLE GET DIABETES?

TREATING DIABETES

A NOTE OF CAUTION

LOW-FAT AND LOW G.I. SNACK FOODS

HYPOGLYCAEMIA — THE EXCEPTION TO THE LOW G.I. RULE

DIABETES COMPLICATIONS

PREVENTING DIABETES

SYNDROME X

●

The G.I. factor has far-reaching implications for diabetes. Not only is it important in treating people with diabetes, but it may also help prevent people from getting diabetes in the first place and possibly even prevent some of the complications of diabetes.

■■■ WHAT IS DIABETES?

Diabetes is a chronic condition in which there is too much sugar or glucose in the blood. Keeping the sugar level normal in the blood needs the right amount of a hormone called **insulin**. Insulin gets the sugar out of the blood and into the body's muscles where it is used to provide energy for the body. If there is not enough insulin or if the insulin does not do its job properly, diabetes develops.

Children and young adults develop diabetes because they cannot make enough insulin. People over the age of 40 usually develop diabetes because their insulin does not work properly. At first the body struggles to make extra insulin because what is there is not working properly; later these people also develop a shortage of insulin. The aim of treatment for people with this type of diabetes is to help them make the best use of the insulin they have and to try to make it last as long as possible.

There are two main types of diabetes:

Type 1, or insulin-dependent diabetes mellitus, occurs most commonly in children and young adults. In this type of diabetes the pancreas does not produce enough insulin and insulin injections are used to supply the deficit; and,

Type 2, or non-insulin-dependent diabetes mellitus, which typically occurs in older adults. These people are usually overweight and their insulin does not work properly. Tablets or insulin injections may be necessary to treat this type of diabetes.

Diabetes is on its way to becoming one of the most common health problems in the world by the year 2000. Currently, in many developing and newly industrialised nations, there is an epidemic of diabetes. Already in some countries half of the adult population has diabetes. It is very common in Australia's Aboriginal people in whom up to one in four has diabetes.

■■■■ WHY DO PEOPLE GET DIABETES?

As we said, the most common type of diabetes is the result of insulin not working properly and it usually affects people over the age of 40. Overeating, being overweight and not exercising enough are important factors (what we call lifestyle factors) which can lead to this type of diabetes, especially when there is someone else in the family with diabetes.

Many people who live in societies which are undergoing rapid westernisation are developing this type of diabetes. Why ?

To find the answer we need to look back in time. Our ancestors lived and evolved in a very cold climate. Over the last 700 000 years there have been many ice ages — the last ended only 10 000 years ago. During these ice ages there was very little plant food around and people had to hunt animals for survival. This gave them a lot of protein in their diet. In other words, during the ice ages our ancestors were carnivores (meat eaters). Their bodies adapted to this way of life to help them survive on this diet — and also to help them survive times when food was scarce.

As it turned out, this protein-based diet would also have protected them from developing diabetes. This is because the main way the body copes when there is not much carbohydrate (glucose) in the diet, is to make sure that the important parts, such as the brain, get what little glucose there is available. To do this the body makes very little insulin, because the brain can use glucose without insulin. Thus the body's insulin supplies are not used up.

Since the end of the last ice age there have been many changes to the type and amount of food that we eat. First, our ancestors began to grow food crops. Agriculture changed their eating pattern from one based on animal protein to one based on carbohydrate in the form of whole cereal grains, vegetables and beans. A dietary change like this would also have changed the sugar levels in their blood. While they ate a high protein diet, the sugar levels in their blood would not have risen significantly after a meal. When they starting eating carbohydrate regularly, the blood sugar level would have increased after meals. The amount by which the sugar levels in the blood increase after a meal depends on the G.I. factor of the carbohydrate. Crops such as wheat grain, which our ancestors grew, have a low G.I. factor. They would not have caused much change in blood sugar levels, so there would have been no need to use up much insulin, either.

The second major change came with industrialisation and the advent of high speed steel roller mills. Instead of eating whole grain products, the new milling procedures broke up the grain into small particles; in fact it enabled us to produce flour so fine it resembled talcum powder. The end result was highly refined carbohydrate. We now know that breaking up natural grain seeds by milling leads to an increase in the G.I. factor of a food, and transforms a low G.I. food into one with a high G.I. factor. When this highly refined food is eaten it causes a greater increase in blood sugar levels. To keep the blood sugar levels normal, the body has to make large amounts of insulin. Many of the commercially packaged foods and drinks with which we now fill our shopping trolleys, have a high G.I. factor. All this strains the body's insulin supplies.

Thirdly, the dramatic increase over the past 50 years in the quantity of high fat takeaway and fast foods that we regularly eat has made matters even worse. So to our already high G.I. foods, we have added a lot of fat as well. As explained in Chapter 5, eating a lot of fat will increase body weight, which in turn makes it harder for the insulin to clear the glucose from the blood. In other words the body becomes insulin resistant — resistant to the effect of insulin. Continually eating carbohydrate foods with a high G.I. factor places even more pressure on the body's ability to keep producing large amounts of insulin to control the blood sugar levels. Add to this insulin resistance, and you have the perfect recipe for eventually exhausting the body's insulin supply and developing diabetes.

It takes time for our bodies to adapt to such major changes in diet. Because, in Europe, our ancestors had thousands of years to adapt to a diet with a lot of carbohydrate, they were in a better position to cope with the changes in the G.I. factor of foods. That is why people of European extraction have a lower prevalence of Type 2 diabetes compared with others, such as Australian Aboriginal people, whose diets have recently changed to include lots of high G.I. foods.

However, there is only so much that our bodies can take. As we continue to consume increasing quantities of foods with a high G.I. factor plus excessive amounts of fatty foods, our bodies are coping less well. The result can be seen as a significant increase in the number of people developing diabetes.

But, the most dramatic increases in diabetes have occurred in populations which have been exposed to these changes over a very much shorter period of time. In some Australian Aboriginal communities up to one person in four now has diabetes. In some groups of native American Indians and in some populations within the Pacific region, up to one adult in two has diabetes because of the rapid dietary and lifestyle changes in the twentieth century. Northern Europeans took around 10 000 years to reach the same point!

▩ TREATING DIABETES

Taking care with what you eat is essential if you have diabetes. For some people, this is all they have to do to keep their blood sugar levels in the normal range of between 4 and 8 millimoles per litre. Others also need to take tablets or injections of insulin. But no matter what the treatment, everyone with diabetes must take care with their food in order to keep their blood sugar levels under control. Keeping the blood sugar near the normal range helps prevent complications of diabetes such as blindness, heart attacks, kidney failure and amputations.

For over a hundred years, people with diabetes have been given advice on what to eat. Many diets were based more on unproven (although seemingly logical) theories, rather than actual research. In 1915, for example, the *Boston Medical and Surgical Journal* advocated that the best dietary treatment for someone with diabetes was 'limitation of all components of the diet'. This translated to a very low kilocalorie diet interspersed with days of fasting. Unfortunately, malnutrition was often the result!

In the 1920s doctors began recommending high fat diets for their patients. Ignorant of the dangers of a high fat diet, they knew that fat, at least, didn't break down to become blood sugar. We now know that high fat diets only hastened the development of heart disease, the most frequent cause of death among people with diabetes.

It was not until the 1970s that carbohydrate was considered to be a valuable part of the diabetic diet. Researchers found that not only did the nutritional status of patients improve with a higher carbohydrate intake, but their blood sugar levels improved as well. The emphasis through the 1970s and for much of the 1980s was on the quantity of carbohydrate in the diet. 'Portion' diets were used to prescribe a set amount of carbohydrate to be eaten at every meal. (A 'carbohydrate portion' was an amount of carbohydrate-rich food which contained 10 to 15 grams of carbohydrate — depending on which country you lived in. So, not only was the portion system complicated, portion sizes varied throughout the world!)

An underlying assumption of the carbohydrate portions theory was that equivalent **amounts** of carbohydrate, irrespective of the **type**, cause an equal change in the blood sugar level. This reasoning had no scientific backing and has since clearly been shown to be incorrect. Fortunately, good quality scientific research supports today's dietary recommendations for people with diabetes. Whilst the G.I. factor research has not negated the significance of the quantity of carbohydrate in the diet, it has shown us the importance of considering the **type** of carbohydrate food that we include.

The only part of food which directly affects blood sugar levels is carbohydrate. When we eat carbohydrate foods, they are broken down into sugar and cause the blood sugar levels to rise. The body responds by releasing insulin into the blood. The insulin clears the sugar from the blood, moving it into the muscles where it is used for energy, so the blood sugar level returns to normal.

Some people think that because carbohydrate raises the blood sugar level, it should not be eaten at all by people who have diabetes. This is not correct. Carbohydrate is a normal part of the diet and at least half of our total daily kilocalories should come from carbohydrate. In fact, the more carbohydrate you eat the better because it automatically reduces the proportion of fat in your diet. **The secret to the diabetic diet is not so much the quantity but the type of carbohydrate.**

Traditionally sugar was excluded from diabetic diets because it was thought to be the worst type of carbohydrate. The simple structure of sugar supposedly made it more rapidly digested and absorbed than other types of carbohydrate, like starch. This assumption was simply not correct. Even in the late 1970s, test meal studies showed that there was a great deal of overlap between the blood sugar responses to sugary and starchy foods. Fifty grams of carbohydrate eaten as potato caused a similar rise in blood sugar to the same amount of sugar. Ice cream resulted in a lower blood sugar response than potato! Findings like these sparked research into the G.I. factor in an effort to learn more about how the body actually responds to different carbohydrate foods.

The G.I. factor has shown us that the way to increase the quantity of carbohydrate in the diabetic diet, without increasing the sugar levels in the blood, is to choose carbohydrate foods with a low G.I. factor.

....

At 50 years of age, Helen had tried many times to lose weight. Her neighbours had started walking on a regular basis but she felt tired all the time and had no energy to do anything more than what she had to. Being 95 kilograms (15 stone) and only 168 centimetres (5 feet 6 inches) tall ruined her morale. Her mother had diabetes and she knew being overweight put her at greater risk, but every time she lost weight she ended up regaining it. Finally, it was no surprise to her when she was diagnosed with diabetes. In fact it was some relief; here at last was a reason for her tiredness.

On her doctor's suggestion, Helen saw a dietitian for help with her diet. At first glance what Helen was eating appeared reasonable. Breakfast was a slice of wholemeal toast or a wholemeal cracker with margarine and black tea. Lunch was a light meal such as celery, lettuce, a slice of cheese, a slice of cold meat, an egg and a couple of crackers, spread with margarine. For dinner she was having soup and a piece of steak with vegetables. She limited herself to a small cocktail potato. The meal was finished by a piece of fruit.

A closer look at her food record showed that Helen's diet was in fact poorly balanced. It was dominated by protein and fat foods and contained insufficient carbohydrate. It didn't contain enough food to provide a good range of nutrients. What's more, Helen herself was struggling with it and often felt hungry since she had cut lollies and biscuits out of her diet.

To improve things, we first looked at the frequency of eating. Helen kept to three meals a day because she had been brought up to believe that was better for her. She agreed to trying a small snack of fruit or a slice of bread between meals. Even though she wasn't on medication for diabetes, the effect of spreading her food intake more evenly across the day, between small meals and snacks, could help to stabilise her blood sugar level and help her lose weight.

We then revised the amount of carbohydrate that she ate, and listed a range of low G.I. carbohydrate foods that were to be her **first priority** at each meal. The filling value of the carbohydrate left her with less space for the proteins that used to dominate her diet. Helen's new diet looked more like this:

Breakfast began with a fresh orange, juiced, and a bowl of oats with sultanas and low-fat milk. Helen added a slice of whole grain bread or raisin toast if she was still hungry.

Lunch was usually a sandwich on whole grain bread with a slice of lean meat and salad and a piece of fruit or a muffin to finish. Sometimes she had vegetable soup or pasta with a vegetable sauce and salad.

The proportion of foods on her **dinner** plate was rearranged, shrinking in the meat department and filling out on the vegetable side. She began to think of carbohydrate food as the basis of the meal and varied between pasta, rice and potato. Twice a week she made a vegetarian dish with legumes like a minestrone soup or a vegetable lasagne. An evening snack was usually a yoghurt or fruit.

After a month on her new eating plan Helen felt better — in fact she felt well enough to tackle some exercise. Taking a serious look at her day, she decided to commit the half hour after dinner to a walk, five nights a week.

Over the next six months Helen's weight dropped from 95 kilograms (15 stone) to 80 kilograms (12½ stone). Her blood sugar levels were mainly within the normal range. She no longer struggled with hunger and felt good about the food she was eating.

Lowering the G.I. factor of your diet as Helen did is not as hard as it seems, because just about every carbohydrate food that you eat has an equivalent food with a low G.I. factor. Our research has shown that blood sugar levels in people with diabetes are greatly improved if foods with a low G.I. factor are substituted for high G.I. factor foods.

We studied a group of people with diabetes and taught them how to alter their diet by substituting the high G.I. foods they were normally eating for carbohydrate foods with a low G.I. factor. After three months, there was a significant fall in their blood sugar levels. They did not find the diet at all difficult and in fact commented on how easy it had been to make the change and how much more variety had been introduced to their diet.

SUBSTITUTING LOW G.I. FOODS FOR HIGH G.I. FOODS — WHAT TO CHANGE

High G.I. Food	Low G.I. Alternative
Bread, wholemeal or white	Bread containing a lot of whole grains
Processed breakfast cereal	Unrefined cereal such as oats or check the G.I. list for processed cereals with a low G.I. factor e.g. Sultana Bran™
Plain biscuits and crackers	Biscuits made with dried fruit and whole grains such as oats
Cakes and muffins	Look for those made with fruit, oats, whole grains
Tropical fruits such as bananas	Temperate climate fruits such as apples and stone fruit
Potato	Substitute occasionally with pasta or legumes
Rice	Try Basmati rice

— and check the G.I. list at the back of the book for lots more low G.I. alternatives.

So, making this type of change in the everyday diet does not mean that the diet has to be restrictive or impossible to eat. There are lots of recipes in this book that can help you reduce the G.I. factor of your diet. The following case history is an example of the results you could obtain.

Bill, a 62-year-old man, was taking every care with his diabetes. He had changed his diet by reducing his total food intake, had lost weight and was exercising regularly. He was doing finger-prick blood sugar level tests at home. Despite his best efforts, he could not achieve a blood sugar level in the desired range of below 8 millimoles/litre after breakfast. At first glance he was eating what most dietitians would consider to be a good breakfast for someone with diabetes: 2 Weetabix with 250 ml /9 fl oz) milk plus 2 slices of wholemeal toast with a scrape of margarine. However, his blood sugar after breakfast was consistently around 11 millimoles/litre. He was advised to make one simple change — to lower the G.I. factor of the carbohydrate by changing the Weetabix to a bowl of rolled oats. This had an immediate impact and his sugar levels after breakfast fell to 7 millimoles/litre.

If you are having trouble controlling your blood sugar level after a meal look up the G.I. factor for the carbohydrates it contains. See if you can find substitutes with a lower G.I. factor amongst the list. Eating a meal with a lower G.I. factor can lower the blood sugar rise after the meal.

Although we haven't mentioned them yet, don't think that fatty foods are not important. They are, especially in people who are overweight. But fatty foods do not increase the sugar levels. Only carbohydrate foods do. However, being overweight and eating fatty foods **prevents** the body's insulin from doing its job and indirectly causes the blood sugar levels to rise. So, eating hot chips or fried rice (mixtures of high G.I. carbohydrate and fat) causes double trouble. Not only does the high G.I. factor of potato and rice increase the blood sugar levels, but the extra fat will also eventually stop the body's insulin from working properly and makes it less effective in clearing the sugar from the blood. Persistently high blood sugar levels will ultimately damage the body.

The G.I. factor is especially important when carbohydrate is eaten by itself and not as part of a mixed meal. Carbohydrate tends to have a stronger effect on our blood sugar level when it is eaten alone. This is the case with between-meal snacks which most people with diabetes have to have. When choosing a between-meal snack, pick one with a low G.I. factor. For example, an apple with a G.I. factor of 36 is better than a slice of soft white bread with a G.I. factor of around 70, and will result in less of a jump in the blood sugar level.

▅▅▅▅ A NOTE OF CAUTION

Some snack foods with a very low G.I. factor (such as peanuts with a G.I. factor of 14) have a very high fat content and are not recommended for people with a weight problem. As an occasional snack they are fine (especially as their fat is monounsaturated), but not every day. Peanuts are also very moreish and it is hard to stop at just one handful!

▅▅▅▅ LOW-FAT AND LOW G.I. SNACK FOODS

Raisin toast
Low-fat milkshake or smoothie
Apple
Low-fat fruit yoghurt
Dried apricots
Peaches and plums
Baked beans
Orange

....

Leanne was seven and a half months' pregnant when she developed gestational diabetes. Her doctor advised her to keep her blood sugar level after meals at less than 7 millimoles/litre.

To check this, Leanne performed finger-prick blood tests on herself every day. The only time she found her blood sugar tended to be higher than 7 was after her main meal in the evening. By looking back over the results of her home blood sugar monitoring, she found that her blood sugar was high if she ate potato but fine when she had pasta. The secret to good blood sugars for Leanne? Pasta more often, and inclusion of low G.I. carbohydrate whenever she had potato.

Many people with diabetes have to resort to tablets to control blood sugar levels because they are unable to cope with the dietary changes suggested. In fact, eating low G.I. carbohydrate foods allows people to eat more and still lose weight because of their effect on satiety, that is the feeling of fullness after eating. The following story shows how you might be able to decrease or stop taking diabetes tablets simply by concentrating on increasing your intake of low G.I. carbohydrate foods.

Mary, 65 years old, was found to have diabetes two years ago. She was overweight and was told that she had to lose several pounds. Although she had been trying to do this before she developed diabetes, she had been unsuccessful. Now she felt that the extra burden of diabetes would make life impossible for her and that she could not do any more than she was already doing with her diet. Because her blood sugar levels were too high she started taking tablets.

When we looked at what Mary ate, we could see that indeed she really was trying hard and was not overeating. However, almost all of her carbohydrate foods had a high G.I. factor. For example, she was having Weetabix or cornflakes for breakfast, morning coffee biscuits for mid-meal snacks, lots of rice with her lunch and evening meals and watermelon was a favourite fruit. All these foods have a high G.I. factor. By changing to All-Bran™ or untoasted muesli for breakfast, having oatmeal biscuits or apples, pears or oranges for snacks and pasta with her main meals, Mary was able to eat more, lose weight and improve her blood sugar levels. Eventually she was able to stop her diabetes tablets too.

■■■ HYPOGLYCAEMIA — THE EXCEPTION TO THE LOW G.I. RULE

In people with diabetes who are treated with insulin or tablets the blood sugar may sometimes fall below 4 millimoles per litre which is the lower end of the normal range. When this happens they might feel hungry, shaky, sweaty and be unable to think clearly. This is called a hypo (short for 'hypoglycaemia').

A hypo is a potentially dangerous situation and must be treated straight away by eating some carbohydrate food. In this case you should pick a carbohydrate with a high G.I. factor because you need to increase your blood sugar quickly. Jelly beans (with a G.I. factor of 80) are a good choice. If you are not due for your next meal or snack you should also have some low G.I. carbohdyrate, like an apple, to keep your blood sugar from falling again until you next eat.

Hypos in the night were a particularly worrying problem for Jane. Her evening insulin doses had been adjusted in an effort to stop her blood sugar going too low at night, but she believed experimenting with her supper carbohydrate could also help. After trying all sorts of different foods and many 3 am blood tests, she struck the answer that the G.I. factor predicted would work — milk! Jane found that a large glass of milk before going to bed, rather than her usual plain biscuits, was easy to drink, and maintained her blood sugar at a good level through the night.

▬▬ DIABETES COMPLICATIONS

If blood sugar levels are not properly controlled, diabetes can cause damage to the blood vessels in the heart, legs, brain, eyes and kidneys. For this reason, heart attacks, strokes, kidney failure and blindness are more common in people with diabetes. It can also damage the nerves in the feet causing pain and irritation in the feet and numbness and loss of sensation.

Many researchers believe that high levels of insulin also contribute to the damage of the blood vessels of the heart, legs and brain. High insulin levels are thought to be one of the factors which might stimulate the muscle in the wall of the blood vessels to thicken. Thickening of the muscle wall causes the blood vessels to narrow and can slow the flow of blood to the point that a clot can form and stop the blood flow altogether. This is what happens to cause a heart attack or stroke.

We know that foods with a high G.I. factor cause the body to produce larger amounts of insulin, resulting in higher levels of insulin in the blood. Therefore, for people with Type 2 diabetes, it makes sense that eating foods with a low G.I. factor will have the effect of helping to control blood sugar levels, and will do this with lower levels of insulin. This may have the added benefit of reducing the large vessel damage which accounts for so many of the problems that diabetes can cause.

▬▬ PREVENTING DIABETES

Most people who develop Type 2 diabetes have a tendency to be unable to produce enough insulin to control their blood sugar levels. Remember, high G.I. foods increase the amount of insulin the body needs, so, for those people susceptible to diabetes, eating carbohydrate with a high G.I. factor will only increase the demand on their already struggling pancreas.

Who is likely to be at risk? People who are over the age of 50, have a family history of diabetes, are overweight, have high blood pressure or have had diabetes during pregnancy (gestational diabetes) are at risk of developing Type 2 diabetes. A reduction of the G.I. factor of their diet could reduce the demand on their pancreas to produce more insulin, perhaps prolonging its function and delaying the development of diabetes. Recent scientific work in the USA has shown quite clearly that those who followed a low G.I. diet had a reduced risk of developing diabetes in later life.

If you fit into one of these categories, you can reduce your chances of getting diabetes by controlling your weight, exercising more and eating more foods with a low G.I. factor.

■■■■ SYNDROME X

Over the past ten years it has become apparent that a number of health problems which cause heart attacks are found together in many people. These include high blood sugar levels, high blood fat levels (especially triglycerides), overweight, high blood pressure and increased blood clotting. When these are found together they are referred to as Syndrome X.

The underlying problem in people with Syndrome X is high levels of insulin in the blood. There are a number of ways that high insulin levels can cause high blood pressure.

High insulin levels in the blood after eating are the result of the carbohydrate in the food. As we have shown before, the high G.I. factor foods cause much higher insulin levels than low G.I. factor foods. One way of controlling the high insulin levels in the blood is to eat low G.I. factor foods. Such a diet will help correct many of the problems found in Syndrome X.

■■■■ A WORD OF ADVICE

There are many factors that can affect your blood sugar levels. If you have diabetes and you are struggling to control your blood sugar level it is important to seek medical help. How much exercise you do, your weight, stress levels, total dietary intake and need for medication may have to be assessed.

CHAPTER 8

THE G.I. FACTOR AND HYPOGLYCAEMIA

TREATING HYPOGLYCAEMIA

•

Hypoglycaemia is a condition in which the sugar level in the blood falls below normal levels. From the Greek words *hypo* meaning under and *glycaemia* meaning blood sugar — hence blood sugar level below normal.

These days, hypoglycaemia is a popular diagnosis for all sorts of problems which cannot be attributed to a more specific diagnosis. There has been considerable publicity about hypoglycaemia which is often blamed for many non-specific health problems ranging from tiredness to depression. Unfortunately, it is often wrongly blamed, which can delay a proper diagnosis and correct treatment.

Nevertheless, genuine hypoglycaemia does occur in a few people, and the G.I. factor has a role to play in treating some forms of this condition. The most common form of hypoglycaemia occurs after a meal is eaten. This is called **reactive hypoglycaemia**.

Normally, when a meal containing carbohydrate is eaten, the blood sugar level rises. This causes the pancreas to make insulin which 'pushes' the sugar out of the blood and into the muscles where it provides energy for you to carry out your regular tasks and activities. The movement of sugar out of the blood and into the muscles is finely controlled by just the right amount of insulin to drop the sugar back to normal. In some people, the blood sugar level rises too quickly after eating and causes an **excessive** amount of insulin to be released. This draws too much sugar out of the blood and causes the blood sugar level to fall below normal. The result is hypoglycaemia.

Hypoglycaemia causes a variety of unpleasant symptoms. Many of these are stress-like symptoms such as sweating, tremor, anxiety, palpitations and weakness. Others affect mental function and lead to restlessness, irritability, poor concentration, lethargy and drowsiness.

The diagnosis of true reactive hypoglycaemia cannot be made on the basis of vague symptoms. It depends on detecting a low blood sugar level when the symptoms are actually being experienced. This means a blood test.

Because it may be difficult (or almost impossible) for someone to be in the right place at the right time to have a blood sample taken while experiencing the symptoms, a glucose tolerance test is sometimes used to try to make the diagnosis. This involves drinking pure glucose which causes the blood sugar levels to rise. If too much insulin is produced in response, a person with reactive hypoglycaemia will experience an excessive fall in their blood sugar level. Sounds simple enough, but there are pitfalls.

Testing must be done under strictly controlled conditions and capillary (not venous) blood samples collected correctly. Home blood glucose meters are not sufficient for the diagnosis of hypoglycaemia.

■■■■■ TREATING HYPOGLYCAEMIA

The aim of treating reactive hypoglycaemia is to prevent sudden large increases in blood sugar levels. If the blood sugar level can be prevented from increasing quickly, then excessive unnecessary amounts of insulin will not be produced and the blood sugar levels will not plunge abnormally low.

Smooth steady blood sugar levels can be readily achieved by changing from high to low G.I. foods in the diet. This is particularly important when eating carbohydrate foods by themselves. Low G.I. foods like whole grain bread, low-fat yoghurt and low G.I. fruits are best for snacks.

If you can stop the big swings in blood glucose levels, then you will not get the symptoms of reactive hypoglycaemia and chances are you will feel a lot better.

Hypoglycaemia due to a serious medical problem is rare. Such conditions require in-depth investigation and treatment of the underlying cause.

TO PREVENT HYPOGLYCAEMIA REMEMBER TO:

■ Eat regular meals and snacks — plan to eat every three hours or so

■ Include low G.I. carbohydrate foods at every meal and for snacks

■ Mix high G.I. foods with low G.I. foods in your meals — the combination will give an overall intermediate G.I.

■ Avoid eating high G.I. foods on their own for snacks — this can trigger hypoglycaemia

An irregular eating pattern is the most common dietary habit that we see in people who have hypoglycaemia. The following case study illustrates this very well.

Diane, with her hectic working life, often did not find time for proper meals. Finally, her body no longer accepted the strain it was under. Diane began to experience odd bouts of weakness and shakiness where she was unable to think clearly. A visit to the doctor and a glucose tolerance test confirmed that she was suffering from hypoglycaemia. The treatment was to change her habits — her eating pattern at least. Diane needed to eat regular meals a day with snacks in between. The thought of eating six times every day seemed an enormous task to Diane — and it took much thought and planning to organise her new diet. What kept her going was how much better she felt almost immediately. The following meal plan is a typical menu for Diane's day.

Breakfast 6 am	Banana, milk, yoghurt, honey and vanilla blended into a smoothie for a speedy start to the day
At work 8.30 am	An oatbran and apple muffin (home-made on the weekend and frozen individually)
Lunch 12 noon	(New habit — must have every day) A substantial sandwich or roll. Occasionally a Mexican dish with beans or a pasta meal if out.
At work 3 pm	Handful of dried fruit (kept in jar in office)
Still at work 5 pm	Couple of oatmeal biscuits (kept in office) for late days
Dinner 7.30 pm	Something quick, often pasta, baked beans on toast or meat and vegetables. (Always double check for carbohydrate in the main) Fruit or milkshake for dessert or late night snack

CHAPTER 9

THE G.I. FACTOR AND RISK OF HEART DISEASE

WHAT IS HEART DISEASE?

WHY DO PEOPLE GET HEART DISEASE?

RISK FACTORS FOR HEART DISEASE

TREATING HEART DISEASE AND SECONDARY PREVENTION

PREVENTING HEART DISEASE: PRIMARY PREVENTION

THE GLYCAEMIC INDEX AND HEART DISEASE

THE GLYCAEMIC INDEX AND INSULIN SENSITIVITY

●

The G.I. factor is important in heart disease too. It has a role in the diets of people who already have heart disease, but perhaps of greater significance in the long term, it has a role in the prevention of heart disease.

WHAT IS HEART DISEASE?

Most heart disease in the Western world, and increasingly elsewhere, is caused by atherosclerosis of the arteries, sometimes referred to as 'hardening of the arteries'. Most people develop atherosclerosis gradually during their lifetime. If it develops sufficiently slowly it may not cause any problems, even into great old age, but if its development is accelerated by one or more of many processes the condition may cause trouble much earlier in life.

Atherosclerosis results in reduced blood flow through the affected arteries. In the heart this can mean that the heart muscle gets insufficient oxygen to provide the power for pumping blood, and it changes in such a way that pain is experienced (central chest pain or angina pectoris). Elsewhere in the body, atherosclerosis has a similar blood-flow reducing effect: in the legs it can cause muscle pains on exercise (intermittent claudication); in the brain it can cause a variety of problems from 'funny turns' to strokes; in the abdomen it can cause poor blood supply to the gut, causing anything from vague 'tummy trouble' to serious malfunction.

An even more serious consequence of atherosclerosis occurs when a blood clot forms over the surface of a patch of atherosclerosis on an artery. This process of thrombosis can result in a complete blockage of the artery with consequences ranging from sudden death to a small heart attack from which the patient recovers quickly. The process of thrombosis can occur elsewhere in the arterial system with a range of consequences determined by the extent of the thrombosis. The probability of developing thrombosis is determined by the 'tendency' of the blood to clot versus the natural ability of the blood to break down clots (fibrinolysis). These two counteracting 'tendencies' are influenced by a number of factors, including some dietary factors (most notably the effect of fatty fish or fish oils in the diet).

People who have gradually developed atherosclerosis of the arteries to the heart (the coronary arteries) may gradually develop reduced heart function. For a while the heart may be able to compensate for the problem, so there may be no symptoms, but eventually it may begin to fail. Shortness of breath may begin to occur, initially on exercise, and there may sometimes be some swelling of the ankles. Modern medicine has many effective drug treatments for heart failure so this consequence of atherosclerosis does not have quite the same serious implications as it did in the past.

■■■■ WHY DO PEOPLE GET HEART DISEASE?

Atherosclerotic heart disease develops early when the many factors that cause it have a strong influence. Over many decades doctors and scientists have identified the processes in fine detail and now most of the factors which cause heart disease are well known. Theoretically this type of heart disease might be largely prevented if everyone's risks were assessed in youth and if all the right things were done throughout the rest of their lives. In practice there has been only a limited development of the ways to screen people for risk early in life, and the resources needed to achieve prevention are just not available. However, a great deal is already being done to identify risk factors in healthy people and those with established heart disease, and those who take the necessary action reduce their risk.

■■■■ RISK FACTORS FOR HEART DISEASE

The chance of developing heart disease is increased if you smoke tobacco, have high blood pressure, have diabetes, have high blood cholesterol (which may be due to eating too much fat in your diet), are overweight or obese and/or do not take enough physical exercise.

■ Smoking of tobacco is now clearly established as a cause of atherosclerosis. Few authorities now dispute the evidence. There are, however, some interesting dietary aspects. Did you know that smokers tend to eat less fruit and vegetables compared to non-smokers (and thus eat less of the protective anti-oxidant plant compounds)? Did you know that smokers tend to eat more fat and more salt than non-smokers? These characteristics of the smoker's diet may be caused by a desire to seek stronger food flavours as a consequence of the taste-blunting effect of smoking. Whilst these dietary differences may make the smoker at greater risk of heart disease there is only one piece of advice for anyone who smokes: **please stop smoking!**

■ High blood pressure causes changes in the walls of the arteries. The muscle layer (remember an artery is not a rigid pipe, it is a muscular tube, which when healthy can change its size to control the flow of blood) becomes thickened and atherosclerosis is more likely to develop. Treatments for blood pressure have become more effective over the last thirty years, but it is only now becoming clear which types of treatment for blood pressure are also effective at reducing heart disease risk.

■ Diabetes is caused by a lack of insulin — either the body does not produce enough or the body 'demands' more than normal (because it has become insensitive to insulin). In diabetes some of the chemical (metabolic) processes which take place tend to accelerate atherosclerosis. Diabetes may also result in raised blood lipids. The increased risk of heart disease is a major reason why so much effort is put into achieving normal control of blood glucose in diabetic patients, and also why all people with diabetes should be checked for the other risk factors of heart disease.

■ High blood cholesterol increases the risk of heart disease. Your blood cholesterol is determined by genetic (inherited) factors — which you cannot change — and lifestyle factors — which you can change. There are some relatively rare conditions in which particularly high blood cholesterol levels occur. People who have inherited these conditions need a thorough 'work-up' by a specialist doctor followed by life-long drug treatment. In most people high blood cholesterol is partly determined by their genes, which have 'set' the cholesterol slightly high, and lifestyle factors which push it up more. The most important dietary factor is fat. The diets prescribed for blood cholesterol lowering are low-fat (low saturated fat), high carbohydrate, high fibre diets. Body weight also affects blood cholesterol — in some people being overweight has a significant effect on the levels — so getting nearer to the ideal weight can be helpful. The blood also contains triglycerides, another type of fat which is particularly high after meals. High triglycerides may be linked with increased risk of heart disease in some people.

■ Overweight and obese people are more likely to have high blood pressure and to have diabetes. They are also at increased risk of getting heart disease. Some of that increased risk is due to the high blood pressure, and the tendency to diabetes, but there is a separate 'independent' effect of the obesity. When increased fatness develops it can be distributed evenly all over the body or it may occur centrally — in and around the abdomen (tummy). This central obesity is particularly strongly associated with the risk of heart disease. Thus every effort should be made to get body weights nearer to normal — especially if the extra weight is 'middle-age spread'.

■ Exercise has several benefits for the heart. Cardiovascular fitness is improved by regular strenuous exercise and the blood supply to the heart may be 'improved'. Exercise is also important in maintaining body weight and has effects on metabolism and some factors related to blood clotting. Getting regular exercise is clearly important.

TREATING HEART DISEASE AND SECONDARY PREVENTION

When heart disease is detected two types of treatment are given. Firstly the effects of the disease are treated (e.g. medical treatment with drugs and surgical treatment to bypass blocked arteries) and, secondly, the risk factors are treated to slow down the further progression of the disease. Treatment of risk factors after the disease has already developed is 'secondary prevention'. In people who have not yet developed the disease, treatment of risk factors is 'primary prevention'. Obviously it would be better to give primary preventive treatment in all cases.

PREVENTING HEART DISEASE: PRIMARY PREVENTION

More and more people now get regular checks of their blood pressure, and sometimes urine tests to check for sugar. Increasingly blood lipid tests are done to check this risk factor too. All health professionals give lifestyle advice on stopping smoking, the benefits of exercise and the nature of a good diet. When specific risk factors are discovered, diet and lifestyle advice is given, but sometimes may not be followed for long. It is especially difficult to follow advice if the effect of not following it is likely not to matter for ten or more years, and if the changes needed are not attractive. The changes must be wanted by the individual who will be helped by encouragement from friends and relatives, and the changes must ideally be positive changes — 'I want to do this' not 'They've told me not to do this.' Any new dimension in heart disease prevention must be seen as a great positive change rather than as a negative.

■■■■ THE GLYCAEMIC INDEX AND HEART DISEASE

The glycaemic index is highly relevant to prevention of heart disease. Since it has benefits for the overweight and those who have diabetes, a low G.I. diet may reduce the risk of heart disease. Blood lipids can also be reduced by low G.I. diets. Those with high blood cholesterol may see a small, but nevertheless useful, reduction of blood cholesterol. It is to be expected that some people will respond more to this dietary change than others and in some cases blood cholesterol reduction may be due to several factors including a reduction in total energy intake, a reduction of fat intake and possibly a reduction of body weight — all occurring from the start of the low G.I. diet. However, the effects of low G.I. diets are not restricted to these effects alone — a further effect has recently been demonstrated.

■■■■ THE GLYCAEMIC INDEX AND INSULIN SENSITIVITY

At the end of Chapter 7 we referred to Syndrome X, a condition char-acterised by high blood sugar levels, high blood fat levels (especially triglycerides), overweight, high blood pressure and increased clotting, all associated with high blood insulin levels. However, there is more to Syndrome X than this — in this condition it is now known that the body is insensitive to insulin. The tissues of the body change so that more insulin is needed to achieve the same effect as usual, and the body responds by circulating more insulin in the blood. Tests on patients with heart disease show that a much higher than expected number of them have this insensitivity to insulin.

Can a low G.I. diet help? In a recent study, patients with serious dis-ease of the coronary arteries were given either low or high G.I. diets before surgery for coronary bypass grafts. They were given blood tests before their diets and just before surgery, and at surgery small pieces of fat tissue were removed for testing. The tests on the fat showed that the low G.I. diets made the tissues of these 'insulin insensitive' patients more sensitive — in fact they were back in the same range as normal 'control' patients after just a few weeks on the diet.

If people with serious heart disease can be improved, would the same happen with younger people? Young women in their thirties were divided into those who did and those who did not have a family history of heart disease. They themselves had not yet developed the condition. They had blood tests followed by low or high G.I. diets for four weeks, after which they had more blood tests, and then when they had surgery (for conditions unrelated to heart disease) pieces of fat were again removed and tested for insulin sensitivity. The young women with a family history of heart disease were insensitive to insulin (those without the family history of heart disease were normal) but after four weeks on the low G.I. diet were normal again.

In both studies the diets were designed to try to ensure that all the other variables (like total energy, total carbohydrate) were not different, so that the change in insulin sensitivity seen was likely to have been due to the low G.I. diet rather than any other factor.

Work on these exciting findings continues but what is known so far strongly suggests that low G.I. diets not only improve body weight and improve blood sugar in people with diabetes, but also improve the sensitivity of the body to insulin. It will take many years of further research to show that this simple dietary change to a low G.I. diet will definitely slow the progress of atherosclerotic heart disease. In the meantime it is clear that risk factors for heart disease are improved by the low G.I. diet. Low G.I. diets are consistent with the other required dietary changes needed for prevention of heart disease. So the message for heart disease prevention is: low fat (low saturated fat), high carbohydrate, high fibre, **low G.I.!**

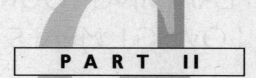

PART II

YOUR GUIDE TO LOW G.I. EATING

PLANNING YOUR LOW G.I. MEALS

....

COOKING THE LOW G.I. WAY

....

THE RECIPES

....

CHAPTER 10

PLANNING YOUR LOW G.I. MEALS

CREATING MEALS TO ACHIEVE THE
G.I. FACTOR YOU NEED

BREAKFAST: USING THE G.I. FACTOR TO
SUSTAIN YOU THROUGH THE DAY

A SIMPLE, HEALTHY LOW G.I. BREAKFAST

QUICK LOW-FAT, LOW G.I. BREAKFAST IDEAS

QUICK LOW-FAT, LOW G.I. BREAKFAST IDEAS

LUNCH: IDEAS FOR A LIGHT MEAL
OR A G.I. LOWERING SIDE DISH

LUNCHING OUT

LOW G.I. LUNCHES ON THE GO

MAIN MEALS: CHOOSING THE BEST WITH LOW G.I.

LOW G.I. DINNER IDEAS

DESSERTS: A LOW G.I. FINISH

QUICK AND EASY LOW G.I. DESSERTS

SNACKS: KEEPING YOUR ENERGY LEVELS UP
BETWEEN MEALS

SUSTAINING SNACKS

▄▄▄ CREATING MEALS TO ACHIEVE THE G.I. FACTOR YOU NEED

Eating a low G.I. diet still means eating a variety of foods. Possibly a wider variety than you are already eating. Potatoes with a high G.I. can still be included. A food is not good or bad on the basis of its G.I. The G.I. factor of a meal consisting of a mixture of carbohydrate foods is a weighted average of the G.I. factors of the carbohydrate foods. The weighting is based on the proportion of the total carbohydrate contributed by each food. Usually we eat a combination of carbohydrate foods, like baked beans on toast, sandwiches and fruit, pasta and bread, cereal and toast, potatoes and corn. Studies show that when a food with a high G.I. factor is combined with a food with a low G.I. factor the complete meal has an intermediate G.I. factor.

Rule of thumb

High G.I. factor food + Low G.I. factor food =

Intermediate G.I. factor meal

Supposing you have a meal of baked beans on toast.

Regular white bread has a G.I. factor of 70,

and baked beans have a G.I. factor of 48.

If we assume half the carbohydrate is coming from the bread, and half from the baked beans, we can add the G.I. factors of the two foods together and divide by 2,

$(70 + 48) \div 2$

giving a final G.I. factor of 59.

So rather than basing the meal on bread alone (a fairly high G.I. factor food) you can lower the G.I. factor of the meal to a more intermediate level by the addition of some low G.I. beans.

The final G.I. factor of a meal depends on the G.I. factors of the foods that make up the meal and the proportion of carbohydrate contributed by each carbohydrate rich food.

If you have two carbohydrate rich foods combined 50:50, you can add their G.I. values and halve the result to come up with the new G.I. factor. But if you have two foods combined in uneven proportions, say ¼ potato : ¾ lentils, then 75 per cent of the G.I. factor of the lentils should be added to 25 per cent of the G.I. factor of potato.

MAKING THE CHANGE TO A LOW G.I. DIET

High G.I. Eating Plan G.I. Factor: 67	Low G.I. Eating Plan G.I. Factor: 41
Breakfast 30 g (1 oz) cornflakes and full cream milk 2 toast (white bread) with margarine and yeast extract	**Breakfast** 30 g (1 oz) Sultana Bran™ and semi-skimmed milk 2 toast (whole grain bread) with margarine and yeast extract An orange
Snack 2 Morning Coffee™ biscuits	**Snack** 2 oatmeal biscuits
Light Meal A sandwich (wholemeal bread) with ham and salad A doughnut	**Light Meal** A sandwich (whole grain bread) with ham and salad Low-fat fruit yoghurt
Snack Piece of watermelon Packet of potato crisps (50 g/2 oz)	**Snack** An apple Small packet (50 g/2 oz) of peanuts (high fat)
Main Meal Lamb Chops Mashed potato Carrots Peas Ice cream and banana	**Main Meal** Small steak Creamy pasta Sweet corn Peas Low-fat ice cream and peaches
Snack Packet of corn chips (40 g/1½ oz)	**Snack** Homemade popcorn (40 g/1½ oz)
Energy value: 2500 kilocalories (10 400 kilojoules) **Fat content:** 120 grams, supplying 44 per cent of energy	**Energy value:** 1800 kilocalories (7500 kilojoules) **Fat content:** 60 grams, supplying 28 per cent of energy

The menu in the right-hand column has a G.I. factor 40 per cent lower than the menu on the left, and its fat content is half that of the high G.I. menu. The quantity of food is similar but the kilocalorie content is nearly one-third lower because low-fat, high carbohydrate foods have been used.

It can be complicated to calculate the precise G.I. factor of a combination of foods unless you have access to food composition figures or a nutrient analysis program. As with kilocalories, the G.I. value is not precise. What G.I. values give you is a guide to lowering the G.I. factor of your day. A simple change can make a big difference. Compare the menus on page 118.

■■■■ BREAKFAST: USING THE G.I. FACTOR TO SUSTAIN YOU THROUGH THE DAY

More and more people these days realise the benefits of having breakfast. Scientifically, having breakfast has been proven to help some people lose weight and to lower their cholesterol levels. We also know that eating breakfast can help to stabilise your blood sugar levels. It kick starts your metabolism and gives your body food when it really needs it. Missing breakfast can cause symptoms of fatigue, dehydration and loss of energy.

One of the things we notice when non-breakfast eaters start having breakfast is that suddenly they develop a morning appetite that they haven't had since childhood. Eating breakfast becomes easier, in fact it becomes a necessity (which is what it should be). Our bodies require fuel to run on and yet too many of us expect to go about our work without topping up our fuel tank first.

If your breakfast leaves you starving by mid morning, have a closer look at what you ate for breakfast. Many breakfast cereals and breads have a high G.I. factor which means whilst they pick you up initially, they won't last long. When the energy runs out and your blood sugar starts to drop, you feel hungry again. Eating a low G.I. breakfast ensures your breakfast is going to take you through to lunchtime.

In the breakfast section you'll find simple recipes from a quick milkshake to delicious mueslis and more adventurous dishes for a weekend breakfast — all guaranteed to sustain you through the day!

■■■■ A SIMPLE, HEALTHY LOW G.I. BREAKFAST

1. Start with some fruit or juice

Fruit contributes fibre and, more importantly, vitamin C, which helps your body absorb the nutrient iron.

LOWEST G.I. FACTOR FRUITS AND JUICES

Cherries	.22	Peaches	.42
Pears	.38	Oranges	.44
Plums	.39	Dried apricots	.31
Apple juice	.40	Pineapple juice	.46
Grapefruit	.25	Apples	.38
Grapes	.46	Grapefruit juice	.48

2. Try some breakfast cereal

Cereals are important as a source of fibre, vitamin B and iron. When choosing processed breakfast cereals, look for those with a high fibre content.

THE TOP FIVE IN LOW G.I. CEREALS

All-Bran™	.42
Sultana Bran™	.52
Special K™*	.54
Muesli	.56
Porridge	.42

(* add some bran to boost its fibre content)

As more research is done and more products are developed, the range of low G.I. cereals will expand.

3. Add milk or yoghurt

Low-fat milks and yoghurts can make a valuable contribution to your daily calcium intake by including them at breakfast. All have a low G.I. factor. Lower-fat varieties have just as much, or more, calcium as full cream milk.

4. Plus some bread or toast if you like

LOWEST G.I. FACTOR BREADS

Pumpernickel	.41
Heavy grain loaf	about 46
Fruit loaf	.47

▇▇▇ QUICK LOW FAT, LOW G.I. BREAKFAST IDEAS

1. Raisin toast spread with fat-reduced cream cheese and topped with sliced apple

2. Porridge sprinkled with raisins and brown sugar

3. A low-fat milkshake

4. A tub of low-fat yoghurt with a sliced peach and raspberries spooned through

5. Bowl of All-Bran™ and low-fat milk, topped with canned pear slices

6. Baked beans on mixed grain loaf with a little avocado

▇▇▇ LUNCH: IDEAS FOR A LIGHT MEAL OR A G.I. LOWERING SIDE DISH

1. Base your light meals on carbohydrate. Foods such as:

Bread	Pasta	Whole grains	Legumes
bread roll	noodles in soup	steamed rice	baked beans
toast	minestrone	sweet corn	mixed bean salad
sandwiches	fettuccine	tabbouli	curried lentils
fruit loaf	pasta salad	rice salad	pea soup
pitta bread	ravioli	savoury rice	chilli beans

2. You might add a little meat, cheese, egg or fish

Simple ideas to add

a sprinkling of Parmesan	hard-boiled egg quarters	slivers of smoked ham
sardines and lemon	chopped cooked chicken	sliced turkey breast
a fold of smoked salmon	a cluster of smoked oysters	a sprinkle of chopped bacon
a smear of pâté	a tub of yoghurt	a cube of cheddar cheese
a slice of pastrami	tuna in brine	sliced roast beef

Remember — keep the quantity small!

3. Fill it out with vegetables

Simple vegetable ideas

fresh salad greens	cherry tomatoes	cucumber	grated carrot
sprouts	a handful of olives	sliced shallots	shredded cabbage
a spoonful of pesto	crunchy celery sticks	whole baby beetroots	tender spinach leaves
a mini pumpkin	whole radish	sun-dried tomatoes	pepper strips
peas	cauliflower chunks	a sliver of ginger	chopped parsley

4. And round it off with fruit

In the Soups, Salads and Pasta recipe section you'll find ideas for quick, low G.I. lunches plus recipes for substantial salads and soups, (both of which can form a superb start for a low G.I. meal).

▄▄▄▄ LUNCHING OUT

We took a look at some lunch time menus and discovered how to make that takeaway lunch a low G.I. choice. Check out the fat content too. Takeaway menu items are often high fat, so we've done our best to put together what can be lower fat options. Of course ingredients and hence fat content varies from place to place, so you need to be reasonably vigilant.

Lunch	Our estimated G.I. factor
Fresh fruit salad with low-fat yoghurt	46 Fat: negligible
Fettuccine with tomatoes, olives and garlic (or any other low-fat sauce you care for)	32 Fat: 8 grams
Go Mexican and choose something with beans, e.g. bean burritos	35 Fat: 11 grams
Stuffed baked potato with baked beans and cheese	72 Fat: 12 grams
Thai noodles with vegetables	36 Fat: 13 grams
A Doner kebab filled with tabbouli, felafel and salad	48 Fat: 21 grams
Charcoal chicken teamed with a small tub of bean salad and a corn cob	39 Fat: 24 grams
or try Indian... a chicken curry with a little dhal and perhaps some Basmati rice	48 Fat: 26 grams

▰▰▰ LOW G.I. LUNCHES ON THE GO

1. Take some pitta bread, spread it with hummus, and fill with tabbouli
2. Chunky vegetable soup, thick with barley, beans and macaroni
   Boil up a bowl of pasta and mix through pesto or chopped fresh herbs
3. Put your favourite sandwich filling on whole grain bread
4. Beat up a banana smoothie and couple it with a high fibre apple muffin
5. Top a tub of fruit salad with a pot of yoghurt
6. Take a green salad plus some bean salad, add grainy bread and enjoy!

■■■ MAIN MEALS: CHOOSING THE BEST WITH LOW G.I.

What to make for dinner is the perennial question. When organising the ingredients in your mind for a main meal, think of them appearing in the following order.

1. First choose the carbohydrate

Which will it be? Potato, rice, pasta, grains, legumes or a combination? Could you add some bread or corn? See below for further help.

Choosing your main meal carbohydrate

It isn't just a matter of choosing the food with the lowest G.I. factor. It is best to include a wide variety of foods in your diet to optimise your nutrient intake. Compare the nutritional properties of these carbohydrate foods and see why variety is important.

Potato	Believe it or not, the potato is a good source of vitamin C and potassium. The content of both these nutrients is higher when less water and shorter cooking times are used in the preparation of potatoes. Potatoes themselves do not contain fat so think twice about how you cook them. Most potatoes have G.I. factors above 60.
Rice	White rice is bland in flavour, making it an ideal accompaniment to spicy Chinese, Thai and Indian food. Milling of rice removes the bran and germ, resulting in a considerable loss of nutrients. Because of this, brown rice is a much better source of B vitamins, minerals and fibre. Vary your diet to include both brown and white rice. The lowest G.I. factor rice is Basmati (at 58).
Sweet potato	Orange sweet potato is a fantastic source of ß-carotene (the plant precursor of vitamin A) and is also quite rich in vitamin C and makes a colourful addition to any dinner. It is a good source of fibre. G.I. factor 54.
Sweet corn	Corn on the cob, or loose kernel corn, is generally a popular vegetable with children and is high in fibre. It is also a source of B vitamins. G.I. factor 55.

Legumes	Chick peas, lentils and beans are all high in protein and so are a nutritious alternative to meat. Their content of niacin, potassium, phosphorus, iron and zinc is also high while their fibre content is higher than for the other carbohydrate foods listed here. G.I. factor varies — check tables at back of book.
Pasta	Pasta is higher in protein than rice or potato and is often eaten as a meal without including meat. It is very satisfying and quick to prepare with the addition of vegetables, or a vegetable sauce and a sprinkling of Parmesan. G.I. factor varies from 37 to 55.
Cracked wheat	Bulgur (burghul) is parboiled whole or cracked grains of wheat. Because the whole grain is virtually intact, bulgur provides lots of fibre, thiamin, niacin, vitamin E and minerals. G.I. factor 48.

2. Add vegetables — and lots of them

Fresh, frozen, canned — whatever you have, the more the merrier. Refer to the vegetables list under lunches for inspiration, or use your favourites. Think of a bowl of crisp salad with a sprinkling of chopped sun-dried tomatoes.

3. Just a little protein for flavour and texture

Remember, we don't need much — some slivers of beef to stir-fry, a sprinkle of tasty cheese, strips of ham, a dollop of ricotta, a tender chicken breast, slices of salmon, a couple of eggs, a handful of nuts, or use the protein found in your grains and legumes.

4. Think twice about using any fat

Check that you are using a healthy type (a monounsaturated or a polyunsaturated) and reduce the quantity if you can.

■■■■ LOW G.I. DINNER IDEAS

1. Team spaghetti Bolognese with a green salad

2. Wrap a fish fillet dressed with herbs, tomato, onion in foil and bake
   Serve with mixed vegetables or salad

3. Make a lasagne — vegetable or beef with salad
   (See the recipes for a low-fat version)

4. Grill a steak and serve with a trio of low G.I. vegetables —
   potato, sweet corn, peas and sweet potato

5. Spicy Lentils and Rice (see recipes)

6. Stir-fry chicken, meat or fish with mixed green vegetables
   Serve with Basmati rice or Chinese noodles

7. Cook spinach and ricotta tortellini with garden vegetables

8. Buy a barbecued chicken, steam sweet corn cobs and toss
   a salad together

9. Taco mix of half mince and half red beans served in a soft
   tortilla bread

■■■■ DESSERTS: A LOW G.I. FINISH

It's fairly easy to give a meal a low G.I. twist through dessert. This is
because so many of the basic components of dessert, like fruit and
dairy products, have a low G.I. factor.

In discussions with people about what they eat these days, dessert
is seldom mentioned. With busier lifestyles and concerns about overweight, dessert is conveniently missed. While this appears a positive
change in eliminating unnecessary sugary, fatty kilocalories from the
diet there is a negative side. In many instances desserts can make a
valuable contribution to our daily calcium and vitamin C intake
because they are frequently based on dairy foods and fruits. What's
more, desserts are usually carbohydrate rich which means they help
top up our satiety centre, signifying the completion of eating.

The basis of a perfect dessert — low G.I. fruits and dairy foods
Citrus A winter fruit which is an excellent source of vitamin C. Select
heavy fruit with fine textured glossy skin. Oranges are good as a snack
cut into quarters and frozen. Soak segments of a variety of citrus fruit
in orange juice with a slurp of brandy, scatter with raisins or sultanas
and serve as winter fruit salad.

Cherries A true summer fruit. Choose plump fruit, bright red/black colour on fresh green stems. A bowl of cherries on the table is a lovely dessert to share.

Stone fruits Apricots appear earliest in the season. Choose those with as much golden orange colour, avoiding pale or green fruit. Peaches and nectarines should be just beginning to soften. Fresh sliced peaches or nectarines are delicious with ice cream or yoghurt. Sprinkle fresh peach halves with cinnamon and try them lightly grilled.

Pears and apples At their peak during autumn and winter, but are available all year. Preparation simply involves washing and slicing and they provide the perfect finish to a meal.

Grapes One of the most popular fruits with children because they are so sweet and easy to eat. Grapes do not ripen after harvest so choose bunches with a deep, uniform colour on fresh green stems. Put a bowl on the table after a meal or include them in a fruit salad.

Custard, ice cream and yoghurt Look for low-fat varieties for a cool and creamy treat.

ADD FRUIT TO SWEETEN...

Sugar or sucrose, a common ingredient in traditional desserts, has a G.I. factor of 65. This means that if a recipe contains a lot of sugar, particularly in combination with flour, with a G.I. of around 70, then your final product can't help but have a high G.I. factor. Recipes incorporating fruit for sweetness will have more fibre and a lower G.I. Remember temperate-climate fruits such as apples, pears and stone fruits tend to have the lowest G.I. values.

▰▰▰ QUICK AND EASY
LOW G.I. DESSERTS

1. Low-fat ice cream and strawberries

2. Baked whole apple, stuffed with dried fruit

3. Fruit salad with low-fat yoghurt

4. Make a fruit crumble — top cooked fruit with a crumbled
   mixture of toasted muesli, wheat flakes, a little melted
   butter and honey

5. Slice a firm banana into some low-fat custard

6. Top canned fruit (peaches or pears) with low-fat ice cream
   or low-fat custard

7. Wrap apple, sultanas, currants and spice in a sheet of filo pastry
   (brushed with milk, not fat) and bake as a strudel.

▰▰▰ SNACKS: KEEPING YOUR ENERGY LEVELS
UP BETWEEN MEALS

The fine art of grazing! Hands up all those who thought that sensible
eating meant keeping to three meals a day? Traditionally, there has
been a belief that sensible eating meant sticking to three square meals
a day. Perhaps this stems from images of an erratic eater. You know the
one, the person who skips breakfast making up for it with snacks
during the day and then feasting before sleeping at night — certainly
not the ideal pattern! New evidence suggests that the people who
graze, eating small amounts of food throughout the day at frequent
intervals, may actually be doing themselves a favour.

A recent study which compared people eating a diet of three meals
a day with those who had three meals and three snacks showed that
snacking stimulated the body to use up more energy for metabolism
compared to concentrating the same amount of food into three meals.
It's as if the more fuel you give your body the more it will burn.

Frequent small meals stimulate the metabolic rate.

The problem with grazing is that most snacks turn out to be high fat foods like cakes, chocolate, snack bars, crisps or pastries. Another criticism of grazing has been that for people who eat too much, increasing the number of times that they face food is tempting disaster. Overeating is less likely to occur if the foods eaten are carbohydrate rich and have a low G.I. factor. Using these foods, you will feel satisfied before you have over-consumed!

■■■■ SUSTAINING SNACKS

Try a muffin

A smoothie

Raisin toast

A juicy orange

A mini-can of baked beans

A bowl of Sultana Bran™
   with low-fat milk

A piece of pitta bread and
   yeast extract spread

A small tub of low-fat yoghurt

A sandwich

Dried apricots

A handful of sultanas

A big green apple

Low-fat ice cream in a cone

A pile of popcorn
   (low-fat of course)

CHAPTER 11

COOKING THE LOW G.I. WAY

HOW YOU CAN REDUCE THE G.I. FACTOR OF
RECIPES AND MEALS

THE A TO Z OF REDUCING THE FAT CONTENT
OF A RECIPE

THE LOW G.I. PANTRY

WHAT TO KEEP IN THE REFRIGERATOR AND FREEZER

THE LOW G.I. FOOD GLOSSARY

•

Many of your favourite recipes can be modified to lower their G.I. factor. The first step is to become familiar with the G.I. factor of a range of foods. Take a critical look at your meals and consider how you could reduce the G.I. factor. Perhaps you could try Sultana Bran™ for breakfast instead of cornflakes or Rice Krispies™? At lunch time you could ask for a sandwich made from a bread based on whole grains instead of refined flour. For your evening meal, why not have pasta instead of potato and add some other low G.I. ingredients like legumes, sweet corn or peas?

Changing one ingredient in a recipe can be enough to lower the G.I. factor of the final dish. The more low G.I. food(s) in the recipe the greater the effect and the lower the G.I. If the recipe is based on high G.I. ingredients and you feel it can't be changed, try serving it with some low G.I. accompaniments.

HOW YOU CAN REDUCE THE G.I. FACTOR OF RECIPES AND MEALS

In place of:	Low G.I. alternative
Bread (smooth textured)	Substitute about 50% of the flour with whole or cracked grains. Good commercial brands, containing large amounts of whole grains, are available
Flour	In baked goods, reduce the amount of flour, partially substituting with oat bran, rice bran, or rolled oats
Rice	Try Basmati rice, or pearled barley, quick-cooking wheat, buckwheat, bulgur, couscous, instant noodles
Potato	Sweet potato, Basmati rice, pasta, sweet corn
Sugar	Try apple juice or dried fruit to sweeten. Honey also has a slightly lower G.I.
Bananas, mango, pawpaw, pineapple, melon, and other tropical fruits have higher G.I. factors	Try apples, cherries, grapefruit, oranges, peaches, pears, plums, and other temperate-climate fruits more often or combine with a higher G.I. fruit to get an intermediate G.I. effect

In recipes for	Low G.I. alternative
Soups	Add lentils, barley, split peas, haricot beans and pasta — make a minestrone!
Casseroles	Try substituting kidney beans, borlotti beans or lentils for a portion of the meat. Boosts the fibre and drops the fat too!
Rissoles or meat loaf	Add cooked lentils, canned beans or rolled oats in combination with the minced meat

HOW TO LOWER THE G.I. OF A RECIPE WHILE KEEPING THE NUTRITION HIGH

Take a recipe such as:
Plain Cup Cakes
I egg
250 ml (9 fl oz) milk
110 g (4 oz) sugar
225 g (8 oz) self-raising flour
110 g (4 oz) butter

The bulk of this recipe is flour (a high G.I. ingredient) plus sugar (an ingredient of intermediate G.I. value). The G.I. factor of the recipe is 67.

■ The first step is to reduce the amount of flour, partially substituting with a lower G.I. food, like oat bran.
■ The next step is to see if some of the intermediate G.I. ingredients can be substituted for ingredients with a lower G.I. Sugar can be partially replaced with fruit or fruit juice, for example.
■ The resulting recipe — a combination of high G.I. ingredients with low G.I. ingredients — gives us a product with a lower total G.I. value.

So, putting some changes into place:

(adding low G.I. fruit for flavour and fibre)	I coarsely grated apple
	I egg
	125 ml (4 fl oz) semi-skimmed or skimmed milk
(using foods with a lower G.I. for sweetness)	125 ml (4 fl oz) apple juice
	60 g (2 oz) sultanas
(reducing the amount of flour)	110 g (4 oz) self-raising flour
(substituting oat bran for flour)	60 g (2 oz) unprocessed oat bran
(reduced amount of butter)	60 g (2 oz) margarine

The finished product: Apple Sultana Muffins which are lower in fat, higher in fibre and have a G.I. factor 10 points lower than the original recipe at 59.

....

THE A TO Z OF REDUCING THE FAT CONTENT OF A RECIPE

As we have said constantly throughout this book, it is important to eat a high carbohydrate and low-fat diet. The following practical tips which we have set out in an easy A to Z format will help you reduce the fat content of some of your favourite recipes at the same time as you are lowering their G.I. factor.

Alcohol Although excessive alcohol consumption can be fattening, as an ingredient in a recipe, alcohol itself won't create a high kilocalorie dish. Alcohol evaporates during cooking, so you lose the kilocalories and are left with the flavour. A little wine in a sauce can give a delicious flavour, and sherry in an Asian style marinade is essential.

Bacon Bacon is a valuable ingredient in many dishes because of the flavour it offers. You can make a little bacon go a long way by trimming off all fat and chopping it finely. Lean ham is often a more economical and leaner way to go. In casseroles and soups, a ham or bacon bone imparts a fine flavour without much fat.

Cheese At around 30 per cent fat (23 per cent of this being saturated), cheese can contribute quite a lot of fat to a recipe. Although there are a number of fat-reduced cheeses available, many of these lose a lot in flavour for a small reduction in fat. It is worth comparing fat per 100 grams between brands to find the tastiest one with the lowest fat content. Alternatively, a sprinkle of a grated, very tasty cheese or Parmesan may do the job.

Ricotta and cottage cheeses are low in fat, usually less than 7 per cent fat. Try them as an alternative to butter or margarine on a sandwich. They yield a fraction of the fat. It's worth trying some fresh ricotta from a deli — you may find the texture and flavour more acceptable than that of the ricotta available in tubs in the supermarket. Flavoured cottage cheeses are ideal low-fat toppings for crackers. Try ricotta in lasagne instead of a creamy white sauce.

Cream and sour cream Keep to very small amounts as these are high in saturated fat. A 300 ml container of cream can be poured into ice-cube trays and frozen providing small servings of cream easily when you need it. Adding one ice-cube block (about 20 ml) of cream to a dish adds only 7 grams of fat.

Dried beans, peas and lentils These are all low in fat and very nutritious. Incorporating them in a recipe, perhaps as partial substitution of meat, will lower the fat content of the finished product. Canned beans, chick peas and lentils are now widely available. They are very convenient to use and a great time saver. They are comparable in food value to the dried ones that you soak and cook yourself.

Eggs Be conscious of eggs in a recipe as they can add fat. Sometimes just the beaten egg white can be substituted for the whole egg.

Filo pastry Unlike most other pastry, filo is low in fat. To keep it that way brush between the sheets with skimmed milk instead of melted butter when you prepare it. Look for it in the freezer section of the supermarket with other prepared pastry and use it as a pie topping or a strudel wrap.

Grilling Grill tender cuts of meat, chicken and fish rather than fry. Marinating first will add flavour, moisture and tenderness.

Health food shops Health food shops can be traps for the unwary. Check out the high fat ingredients, such as hydrogenated vegetable oil, nuts, coconut and palm kernel oil in the products such as muesli bars, nut bars, health cakes and pies (even if made with wholemeal flour) that they stock on their shelves.

Ice cream A source of carbohydrate, calcium, riboflavin, retinol and protein and low-fat varieties have the lower G.I. factor — definitely a nutritious and icy treat.

Jam A dollop of jam on toast contains 22 per cent fewer kilocalories than a smear of butter or margarine on toast. So, enjoy your jam and give fat the flick!

Keep jars of minced garlic, chilli or ginger in the refrigerator to spice up your cooking in an instant.

Lemon Try a fresh squeeze with ground black pepper on vegetables rather than a dob of butter.

Milk Many people dislike skimmed milk, particularly when they taste it on its own or in their coffee! However, you can use skimmed milk in a recipe and no one will notice — and the fat saving is great. For convenience you might want to keep powdered skimmed milk in the pantry that can be made up to the desired quantity when you need it. It will taste more like fresh milk if you mix the powder and water according to directions and refrigerate the milk overnight before using it. UHT (long life) milk is handy in the cupboard, too.

Nuts They are valuable for their content of vitamin E, but they are also high in fat. To keep the fat content of a recipe low, the quantity of nuts has to be small.

Oil Most of our recipes call for no more than 2 teaspoons of oil. Any polyunsaturated or monounsaturated oil is suitable. Cooking spray or brushing oil lightly over the base of the pan is ideal. If you find the amount of oil insufficient, cover your pan, or add a few drops of water and use steam to cook the ingredients without burning. It is a good idea to invest in a nonstick frying pan if you don't have one!

Pasta A food to eat more of and a great source of carbohydrate and B vitamins. Fresh or dried, the preparation is easy. Just boil in water until just tender or 'al dente', drain and top with a dollop of pesto, a tomato sauce or a sprinkle of Parmesan and pepper. There are many wonderful pasta cookbooks now available. It is definitely worth investing in one to find all sorts of exciting ways to prepare this fabulous low G.I. food. Pasta may appear in your menu as a side dish to meat, as noodles in soup, as a meal in itself with vegetables or sauce or even as an ingredient in a dessert.

Questions Ask your dietitian for more recipe ideas.

Reduce the fat content of minced meat by browning it in a non-stick pan, then placing the meat in a colander and pouring boiling water through it to wash away the fat. Return to the pan to continue cooking. It is a good idea to buy the better quality minced beef with less fat.

Stock If you are prepared to go to the effort of making your own stock — good for you! Prepare it in advance, refrigerate it then skim off the accumulated fat from the top. Prepared stock is available in long-life cartons in the supermarket. Stock cubes are another alternative. Look for brands that have reduced salt.

To sauté Heat the pan first, brush with the recommended amount of oil or less, add the food and cook, stirring lightly over a gentle heat.

Underlying the need for fat is a need for taste. Be creative with other flavourings.

Variety Varying ingredients creates more possibilities and provides more nutrients. Branch out and try something you've never tasted before.

Weighing What's the weight of the meat you're buying? Start noticing the weight that appears on the butcher's scales and consider how many servings it will give you. With something like steak, that is basically all edible meat, 120 to 150 g (4 to 5½ oz) per serving is sufficient. Half a kilogram (18 oz) is more than enough for four servings. Choose lean cuts of meat. Trim the fat off before cooking or before you put it away. Alternate meat or chicken with fish once or twice a week.

Yoghurt Yoghurt is a valuable food in many ways. It is a good source of calcium, and 'friendly bacteria', protein and riboflavin and, unlike milk, is suitable for those who are lactose intolerant. Low-fat natural yoghurt is a suitable substitute for sour cream. If using yoghurt in a hot sauce or casserole, add it at the last minute and do not let it boil, or it will curdle. It is best if you can bring the yoghurt to room temperature before adding to the hot dish. To do this, mix a small amount of yoghurt with a little sauce from the dish then stir this mixture back into the bulk of the sauce.

Zero fat is unhealthy, so speak with the professionals (dietitians) about how to get just the right amount you need. Fat does add flavour — use it to your advantage.

▬▬▬ THE LOW G.I. PANTRY

To make low G.I. choices, easy choices, you need to keep the right foods in your pantry.

Breads
    Pumpernickel
    Mixed grain loaves
    Fruit loaf (the heavy types. Keep a loaf in the freezer)
Cereals
    All-Bran™ (Kellogg's)
    Sultana Bran™ (Kellogg's)
    Muesli
    Rolled oats
    Oat bran
    Rice bran
    Pearl barley
    Basmati rice
    Pasta of various shapes and flavours
Canned or dried lentils (red and brown), legumes (chick peas, cannellini beans)
A variety of canned legumes (kidney beans, mixed beans, baked beans)

Canned sweet corn. Other canned vegetables like canned tomatoes, asparagus, peas, mushrooms are always handy to boost the vegetable content of a meal

Canned chopped tomatoes and tomato purée, bottled tomato pasta sauces

Prepared chicken stock or stock cubes

Low-oil salad dressings

Dried fruits — sultanas, dried apricots, fruit medley, raisins, prunes etc.

Canned peaches, pears, apple

Long-life skimmed milk or skimmed milk powder

Canned evaporated skimmed milk

Custard powder

Spices — curry powder, cumin, turmeric, mustard etc.

Herbs — oregano, basil, thyme are the most used in these recipes. Pre-mixed blends of these are available

Bottled minced ginger, chilli and garlic

▆▆▆ WHAT TO KEEP IN THE REFRIGERATOR AND FREEZER

Skimmed or semi-skimmed milk

Low-fat natural yoghurt

Low-fat fruit yoghurt

Low-fat ice cream

Frozen low-fat yoghurt, sorbet

Eggs

Cheese
   low-fat processed slices
   fat-reduced or low-fat cheddar
   grated Parmesan
   cottage or ricotta cheese

Frozen peas and corn

Frozen berries

THE LOW G.I. FOOD GLOSSARY

This glossary describes some of the key foods that can form part of a low G.I. diet.

Apples (G.I. of 38) • Easy-to-incorporate into the diet as a low G.I. food — an average apple will add 3 grams of fibre to your diet. They are also high in pectin which lowers their G.I. factor.

Apple juice (G.I. of 40) • The main sugar occurring in apples is fructose (6.5 per cent) which itself has a low G.I. The high concentration of sugars is known to slow the rate of stomach emptying, hence slowing the absorption and lowering G.I.

Apricots (G.I. of 57, fresh; 64, canned; 31, dried) • Apricots are an excellent source of ß-carotene and dried apricots in particular are high in potassium. Like apples, they are high in fructose (5.1 per cent) which lowers their G.I.

Barley (G.I. of 25) • 'Pearled' barley, which has had the outer brown layers removed, is most commonly used. It is high in soluble fibre which probably contributes to its low G.I. Available in supermarkets.

Basmati rice (G.I. of 58) • Has a low G.I. attributable to the type of starch it contains (high amylose starch). Available in supermarkets.

Breakfast cereals • The high degree of cooking and processing of commercial breakfast cereals tends to make the starch in them more rapidly digestible, giving a higher G.I. Less processed cereals (muesli, rolled oats) tend to have lower G.I. values. Sultana Bran™ (G.I. of 52) and All-Bran™ (G.I. of 42) (Kellogg's), although processed, are not made from milled starch but large flakes of raw bran.

Buckwheat (G.I. of 54) • Buckwheat is available from health food stores and some supermarkets. It can be cooked as a porridge or steamed and served with vegetables, in place of rice. It can also be ground and used as flour for making pancakes and pasta. Buckwheat in this form is likely to have a higher G.I. than when whole.

Bulgur (burghul) (G.I. of 48) • Is made by roughly grinding previously cooked and dried wheat. Most commonly recognised as a main ingredient in tabbouli. The intact physical form of the wheat contributes to its low G.I.

Cherries (G.I. of 22) • The G.I. for cherries is based on European cherries. Australian cherries which are 6.1 per cent glucose and 4.2 per cent fructose may have a higher G.I. value.

Custard (G.I. of 43) • Made with milk, so provides calcium, protein and B vitamins plus a little sugar, vanilla flavouring and a starch thickener.

Fruit loaf (G.I. of 47) • Available in wholemeal and white varieties, but choose the heavy types. The G.I. of fruit loaf is probably lowered by part substitution of flour (high G.I.) with fruit (lower G.I.).

Grapefruit (G.I. of 25) • The low G.I. factor of grapefruit may be due to their high acid content which slows absorption from the stomach.

Grapes (G.I. of 46) • An equal mix of fructose and glucose and a high acid content are characteristics of fruits with a low G.I. Grapes are a good example.

Ice cream (G.I. of 61) • Most dairy products have very low G.I. factors. When we eat dairy foods a hard protein curd forms in the stomach and slows down its emptying. This has the effect of slowing down absorption and lowering the G.I. factor.

Kiwifruit (G.I. of 52) • Kiwifruit contain equal proportions of glucose and fructose giving a reasonably low G.I. They are also a wonderful source of vitamin C with one kiwifruit meeting the total recommended daily intake.

Legumes (G.I. range: 14 to 56) • Also known as pulses. These include dried peas, beans and lentils, mostly with a G.I. factor of 50 or less. Canned varieties have a slightly higher G.I. than their home-cooked counterpart due to the higher temperature during processing. Soya beans (G.I. of 18) have one of the lowest G.I. values, possibly due to their higher protein and fat content. The viscous fibre in legumes reduces physical availability of starch to digestive enzymes.

Milk (G.I. of 27) • Lactose, the sugar occurring naturally in milk, is a disaccharide which must be digested into its component sugars before absorption. The two sugars that result, glucose and galactose, compete with each other for absorption. This slows down absorption and lowers the G.I. The presence of protein and fat in milk also lowers the G.I. of milk.

Oat bran (G.I. of 55) • Unprocessed oat bran is available in the cereal section of supermarkets, usually loosely packed in plastic bags. Its carbohydrate content is lower than that of oats and it is higher in fibre, particularly soluble fibre, which is probably responsible for its low

G.I. A soft, bland product, it is useful as a partial substitution for flour in baked goods to lower the G.I.

Oranges (G.I. of 44) • Well known as a good source of vitamin C, most of the sugar content of oranges is sucrose. This, and their high acid content, probably accounts for their low G.I.

Parboiled rice (G.I. range: 38–87) • Parboiling involves steeping rice in hot water and steaming it prior to drying and milling. Nutrients from the bran layer are retained in the grain and the cooked product has less tendency to be sticky. Some studies have found parboiled rice to have a lower G.I. but studies on Australian rice have found only small differences between parboiled and regular rice. The overriding determinant of the G.I. of rice is the type of starch present in the grain.

Pasta (G.I. range: 32–64) • Pasta is made from hard wheat semolina with a high protein content, which gives a strong dough. Protein-starch interactions and minimal disruption to the starch granules during processing contribute to the low G.I. There is some evidence that thicker pasta has a lower G.I. than thin types.

Peach (G.I. of 42, fresh; 30, canned) • Most of the sugar in peaches is sucrose (4.7 per cent). Other aspects like their acid and fibre content may account for their low G.I.

Peanuts (G.I. of 14) • A low carbohydrate but high fat food, being 50 per cent fat and 25 per cent protein, which is one reason for the low G.I. value.

Pear (G.I. of 38, fresh; 44, canned) • Another fruit with a high fructose (6.7 per cent) content, accounting for the low G.I.

Peas (G.I. of 48) • Peas are high in fibre and also higher in protein than most other vegetables. Protein-starch interactions may contribute to their lower G.I. They also average 3.5 per cent sucrose giving them a sweet flavour.

Pineapple juice (G.I. of 46) • Mainly sucrose (7.9 per cent).

Pitta bread (G.I. of 57) • Unleavened flat bread was found to have a slightly lower G.I. than regular bread in a Canadian study. Sold in supermarkets in packets of flat rounds.

Plums (G.I. of 39) • The G.I. for plums comes from a European study. Plums contain a fairly equal mixture of glucose, fructose and sucrose. The higher concentration of sugars, the slower the food is emptied from the stomach and hence the slower the absorption. This may account for the low G.I.

Popcorn (G.I. of 55) • A surprisingly low G.I. for a processed product. The type of starch or changes to its structure in the popping and cooling of the popcorn may be the cause of the lower G.I. Popcorn is a high fibre snack food.

Porridge • Published G.I. factors range from a low 42 up to 66 for 'one minute oats'. The additional cutting of rolled oats to produce quick cooking oats probably increases the rate of digestion causing a higher G.I.

Potato (G.I. range 56–83) • In potatoes the amylose (slowly digested starch) varies with variety. The branching of amylopectin increases as potatoes mature, thus potatoes harvested from August onwards have more highly branched amylopectin and are likely to be more digestible, giving a higher G.I., while new potatoes may have a lower G.I. Boiled potatoes eaten hot are more digestible than boiled potatoes eaten cold. Reheating increases digestibility a little. The lowest G.I. potatoes are likely to be those from the early part of the harvest (new potatoes) and those eaten cold, e.g. as part of cold potato salad.

Pumpernickel bread (G.I. of 41) • Also known as rye kernel bread because the dough it is made from contains 80 to 90 per cent whole rye kernels. It has a strong flavour and is usually sold thinly sliced. Because it is not made with fine flour, its G.I. is much lower than ordinary bread. Available in supermarkets and delicatessens.

Quick-cooking wheat (G.I. of 54) • Whole wheat grains which have been physically treated to allow short cooking times. It is most often used as a substitute for rice. The whole grain structure also acts as a barrier and so reduces its digestibility and hence lowers the G.I.

Rice bran (G.I. of 19) • Rich in fibre (25 per cent by weight) and oil (20 per cent by weight), rice bran has an extremely low G.I.

Spaghetti (G.I. of 41) • While both fresh and dried pastas have a low G.I., this is not the case for canned spaghetti. Canned spaghetti is generally made from flour rather than high protein semolina and is very well cooked — two factors which are likely to give it a high G.I.

Sultanas (G.I. of 56) • Sultanas are less acidic than grapes and this may account for their slightly higher G.I. since increased acidity is associated with lower G.I. factors.

Sweet corn (G.I. of 55) • Fresh, frozen or canned varieties would be suitable to use. Corn on the cob has a lower G.I. than corn chips or cornflakes. The intact whole kernel makes enzymic attack more difficult.

Sweet potato (G.I. of 54) • Belonging to a different plant family to regular potato, sweet potatoes are mainly available either white or yellow/orange in colour. The 'sweetness' comes from a high sucrose content. Sweet potato is high in fibre. It has a lower G.I. than ordinary potato varieties.

Yoghurt (G.I. of 33) • A concentrated milk product, soured by the use of specific bacteria. All varieties have a low G.I, including those containing sugar. Artificially sweetened brands have both a lower G.I. factor and contain fewer kilocalories.

CHAPTER 12

THE RECIPES

BREAKFASTS

SOUPS, SALADS AND PASTAS

MAINS AND ACCOMPANIMENTS

DESSERTS

SNACKS

●

Low G.I. eating means making a move back to the high carbohydrate foods which are staples in many parts of the world. The emphasis is on whole foods like whole grains — barley, oats, dried peas and beans, in combination with certain types of rice, breads, pasta, vegetables and fruits. We have developed and tested over 50 recipes to help you get started.

You'll find the recipes listed under each of our three main eating occasions — breakfasts, light meals (like soups, salads and pastas), and main meals with additional sections on desserts and snacks. While some of the recipes are specifically modified to lower the G.I., others are included to present new ways of preparing low G.I. foods.

The recipes have been developed to help you reduce the overall G.I. factor of your diet, improving its nutritional quality while you do it. They are designed to be incorporated into your usual diet, helping you to get your carbohydrate intake up to 50 to 60 per cent of your energy intake and keeping your fat intake down to the recommended level of 30 per cent of kilocalories per day. The recipes are high in fibre, both soluble and insoluble. Salt has been added where necessary for flavour, but may be omitted according to taste.

Each recipe has been analysed for its nutritional value which is given per serving where the recipe is divided into a specified number of servings. The following information will help put this nutritional profile into context for you.

Kilocalories (kilojoules) This is the measure of how much energy the food provides. Those who burn lots of energy through exercise need a higher kilocalorie intake than those who live more sedentary lives. A moderately active woman aged 18 to 54 years would consume about 2000 kilocalories; a man about 2500 kilocalories.

Fat Our fat requirement is probably as small as 10 grams a day to provide essential fatty acids needed for health. The range of acceptable fat intake depends on your total kilocalorie intake. People trying to lose weight could aim for around 30 to 40 grams of fat a day. Most others could do with 50 to 60 grams. Children and adolescents need more than adults because they are growing and should not have their fat intake restricted excessively.

Carbohydrate The total amount of carbohydrate (which includes starches and sugars) is listed with each recipe. Our aim is to help you increase your carbohydrate intake as your fat intake drops. It is not necessary to calculate how many grams of carbohydrate you eat on a daily basis; however, the athlete or person with diabetes may find this information useful. This is so they can eat enough! On average, women should take in 250 grams of carbohydrate each day whilst men need about 350 grams. Athletes can consume anywhere from 350 to 700 grams of carbohydrate a day.

Dietary Fibre (or Non-Starch Polysaccharide, NSP) It is recommended that we consume at least 18 grams of non-starch polysaccharide every day. A slice of wholemeal bread provides 1.5 grams of NSP, an average apple 2 grams. The average Briton consumes only 12 grams of non-starch polysaccharide a day.

WEIGHTS AND MEASURES

Weights and volumes in the following recipes are given in metric and imperial, with smaller quantities measured using standard teaspoon (5 ml) and tablespoon (15 ml) measuring spoons. All spoon measures are level unless otherwise stated. The conversion of quantities results in cumbersome numbers which have been rounded up or down for ease of use. The *rounded* conversions used in the recipes are generally as follows:

Grams (g)	Ounces (oz)
25	1
40	1½
55	2
85	3
100	3½
115	4 (¼ lb)
125	4½
140	5
150	5½
175	6
200	7
225	8 (½ lb)
250	9
280	10
300	10½
350	12
375	13
400	14
425	15
450	16 (1 lb)
500	18

Millilitres (ml)	Teaspoons (tsp)
5	1
10	2

Millilitres (ml)	Tablespoons (tbsp)
15	1
30	2
45	3

Millilitres (ml)	Fluid ounces (fl oz) and pints (pt)
30	1
60	2
100	3½
125	4
150	5 (¼ pt)
200	7
250	9
300	10 (½ pt)
425	15 (¾ pt)
450	16
500	18
600	20 (1 pt)
750	25 (1¼ pt)
850	30 (1½ pt)
1.2 litres	32 (2 pts)

BREAKFASTS

HONEY BANANA SMOOTHIE

SWISS MUESLI

PORRIDGE WITH BANANA AND RAISINS

FRUIT 'N' OAT HOTCAKES

SPECIAL PANCAKES

QUICK HAM AND BEANS

CRISPY TOAST AND TOMATOES

KEDGEREE

●

HONEY BANANA SMOOTHIE

The 'smoothie' — a quick but sustaining breakfast. Many variations are possible using different combinations of fruits, milks and yoghurts.

•

G.I. FACTOR: 49
NUTRIENTS PER SERVING: 190 kcal (800 kJ)

FAT............................0.5 g
CARBOHYDRATE..........35 g
FIBRE..........................2 g

---

1 large, ripe banana

250 ml (9 fl oz) semi-skimmed milk, chilled

125 ml (4 fl oz) evaporated low-fat milk, well chilled

10 ml (2 teaspoons) honey

few drops vanilla essence

1. Peel banana and chop roughly.

2. Combine with remaining ingredients in a blender and blend for 30 seconds or until smooth and thick.

3. Serve immediately.

SERVES 2

For this recipe the evaporated milk must be chilled to froth up well. Carnation Lite^{TM} is available in large supermarkets.

SWISS MUESLI

*This muesli requires planning the night before but it is
quick and delicious the following morning.*

•

G.I. FACTOR: 56
NUTRIENTS PER SERVING: 367 kcal (1540 kJ)

FAT	11 g
CARBOHYDRATE	50 g
FIBRE	6 g

1. Combine the oats, milk and raisins in a
   bowl. Cover and refrigerate overnight.

2. Add the yoghurt, almonds and apple;
   mix well.

3. To serve, adjust the flavour with lemon
   juice. Serve with fresh fruit and a drizzle
   of cream as a treat.

   SERVES 4

180 g (6 oz) rolled oats

310 ml (½ pt) semi-skimmed
milk

50 g (2 oz) raisins

100 g (3½ oz) low-fat plain
yoghurt

40 g (1½ oz) whole almonds,
chopped

1 apple, grated

lemon juice (optional)

mixed fresh fruit, such as
strawberries, pear, plum,
passionfruit

40 ml (2½ tablespoons) fresh
cream (optional)

*The fat content is a little high for everyday use,
but most of this comes from the nuts which are
high in monounsaturated fat. Use any nuts of
your choice, if preferred.*

PORRIDGE WITH BANANA AND RAISINS

A tasty porridge variation.

•

G.I. FACTOR: 55
NUTRIENTS PER SERVING: 212 kcal (890 kJ)

FAT ....3 g
CARBOHYDRATE..........38 g
FIBRE...........................3 g

60 g (2 oz) rolled oats

250 ml (9 fl oz) semi-skimmed milk, approximately

1 small ripe banana, mashed

30 g (1 oz) raisins

1. Place the oats in a saucepan or large microwave jug. Add sufficient water to cover plus about two-thirds of the milk.

2. Bring to the boil and boil for 2 minutes or microwave (100% power) for 1 to 2 minutes.

3. Add the banana and cook 1 to 2 minutes more.

4. Add the remaining milk to make a smooth consistency and stir through raisins.

SERVES 2

FRUIT 'N' OAT HOTCAKES

Moist, spicy hotcakes, studded with currants.

•

G.I. FACTOR: 59
NUTRIENTS PER HOTCAKE: 93 kcal (390 kJ)

FAT	2 g
CARBOHYDRATE	19 g
FIBRE	2 g

1. Combine the milk and honey in a saucepan or microwave jug and warm until blood temperature (about 50 seconds on 100% power in microwave oven). Remove from heat and sprinkle in the yeast. Mix well with a fork.

2. Combine the rolled oats, bran, currants and sifted flour and spices in a large bowl. Pour in the milk and yeast mixture and stir to combine. Let stand in a warm place for 15 to 30 minutes. Do not stir again. Mixture will increase in volume and thicken on standing.

3. Heat a nonstick frying pan over moderate heat. Spray with cooking spray or lightly grease with margarine. Without stirring, take spoonfuls of oat mixture from the bowl and drop off the spoon into the pan. Cook until browned underneath, then turn and brown on the other side. (This will take about 3 to 4 minutes.)

4. Serve hotcakes immediately with fruit spread or jam.

MAKES 10 HOTCAKES

375 ml (13 fl oz) semi-skimmed milk

10 ml (2 teaspoons) honey

1 x 7 g sachet dry yeast

30 g (1 oz) rolled oats

60 g (2 oz) oat bran

60 g (2 oz) currants

75 g (2½ oz) plain flour

½ teaspoon ground cinnamon

½ teaspoon mixed spice

fruit spread or jam, to serve

SPECIAL PANCAKES

A light pancake with a lower G.I. than your average pancake.
This is achieved by substituting oats or oat bran for some of the flour.

•

G.I. FACTOR: 56
NUTRIENTS PER PANCAKE: 129 kcal (540 kJ)

FAT ....2 g
CARBOHYDRATE..........22 g
FIBRE...........................2 g

*100 g (3½ oz) 1-minute oats or
unprocessed oat bran*

500 ml (18 fl oz) buttermilk

*75 g (2½ oz) dried fruit medley,
chopped*

75 g (2½ oz) plain flour, sifted

2 teaspoons sugar

1 teaspoon bicarbonate of soda

1 egg, lightly beaten

10 g (½ oz) margarine, melted

semi-skimmed milk (optional)

1. Combine the oats and buttermilk in a
   bowl and let stand 10 minutes.

2. Stir in the dried fruit, flour, sugar,
   bicarbonate of soda, egg and margarine;
   mix thoroughly. Let stand for up to
   1 hour.

3. After standing, add a little semi-
   skimmed milk if the mixture is too
   thick.

4. Heat a nonstick frying pan and spray
   with cooking spray or grease lightly
   with margarine. Pour in about 3
   tablespoons of batter, cook over
   moderate–high heat until bubbly on
   top and lightly browned underneath.
   Turn pancake to brown on other side.
   Repeat with remaining batter.

MAKES ABOUT 10
(SMALL) PANCAKES

---

*Dried fruit medley is a mixture of dried fruit and
is available from supermarkets and health food
stores.*

QUICK HAM AND BEANS

*Team baked beans with low G.I. toast for a
substantial breakfast, if desired.*

•

G.I. FACTOR: 39
NUTRIENTS PER SERVING: 138 kcal (580 kJ)

FAT ....5 g
CARBOHYDRATE..........12 g
FIBRE ....5 g

1. Chop the gammon into small dice.
   Brush the base of a saucepan with a
   little oil and heat. Add the gammon and
   cook lightly.

2. Add the baked beans and heat gently.

3. Remove from heat and stir in the cheese.
   Serve on toast, if desired, sprinkled with
   parsley to garnish.

   SERVES 4

2 large slices gammon

420 g (15 oz) can baked beans

*60 g (2 oz) grated low-fat
cheddar cheese*

*1 tablespoon chopped fresh
parsley*

CRISPY TOAST AND TOMATOES

*You can reduce the fat content of this dish by omitting the margarine.
The vegetable mixture itself makes a nice accompaniment to eggs.*

•

G.I. FACTOR: 49
NUTRIENTS PER SERVING: 162 kcal (680 kJ)

FAT ....9 g
CARBOHYDRATE..........15 g
FIBRE............................5 g

5 ml (1 teaspoon) olive oil

1 small leek, washed and finely sliced

5 small (50 g/2 oz) mushrooms, sliced

2 slices low G.I. bread

15 g (½ oz) margarine

½ punnet (about 100 g/3½ oz) cherry tomatoes, halved

2 teaspoons finely chopped fresh basil

1 teaspoon finely chopped fresh oregano

1 teaspoon finely chopped fresh parsley

freshly ground black pepper

1. Heat the oil in a frying pan, add the leek and mushrooms and cook over medium heat for about 4 to 5 minutes or until tender.

2. Meanwhile, spread the bread very lightly on both sides with margarine. Place under a heated grill and toast both sides until golden brown.

3. Add the tomatoes and herbs to the leek mixture and cook for 1 to 2 minutes longer, or until heated through. Season to taste with pepper and serve on the toast.

SERVES 2

KEDGEREE

This is traditionally a breakfast dish, but it could be used as a filling main course.

•

G.I. FACTOR: 58

NUTRIENTS PER SERVING: 340 kcal (1428 kJ)

FAT	11 g
CARBOHYDRATE	34 g
FIBRE	1 g

1. Place the haddock fillets in a saucepan and cover with the water. Bring to the boil, put a lid on the pan and simmer gently for about 8 minutes. Drain off the cooking water into a measuring jug and reserve. Transfer the haddock to a dish, cover and keep warm.

2. Melt two-thirds of the margarine in the saucepan and soften the onion in it for 5 minutes. Stir in the curry powder and cook for 30 seconds, then stir in the rice and add 240 ml (8½ fl oz) of the cooking water. Stir once, bring to a simmer, cover with a tight-fitting lid and cook very gently for 10 minutes or until the grains are tender.

3. When the rice is ready, remove it from the heat. Flake the fish and fork it into the rice with the egg, herbs, lemon juice and the remaining margarine, and season to taste with salt and pepper. Cover the pan with a clean folded tea towel and replace it on a very low heat for 5 minutes. Tip into a hot serving dish.

SERVES 3 (2 as a main course)

300 g (10 oz) smoked haddock fillets, skinned

280 ml (10 fl oz) cold water

30 g (1 oz) polyunsaturated margarine

1 small onion, finely chopped

¼ teaspoon medium-hot curry powder

120 g (4 oz) long grain rice (Basmati)

1 large egg, hard-boiled, peeled and chopped

1 heaped teaspoon chopped fresh parsley

1 dessertspoon chopped fresh chives

10 ml (2 teaspoons) lemon juice

salt and pepper

SOUPS, SALADS AND PASTAS

TASTY TOMATO AND BASIL SOUP

LENTIL SOUP

MINESTRONE

SPLIT PEA SOUP

MUSHROOM AND CRACKED WHEAT SALAD

PASTA AND BEAN SALAD

RED BEAN SALAD

ITALIAN BEAN SALAD

PASTA AND LENTIL SALAD

TABBOULI

BACON, BEANS AND PASTA IN TOMATO SAUCE

VEGETABLE LASAGNE

CREAMY MUSHROOMS AND PASTA

FETTUCCINE WITH BACON AND MUSHROOM SAUCE

●

TASTY TOMATO AND BASIL SOUP

A delicious variation on tomato soup, with a secret ingredient of sweet potato.

•

G.I. FACTOR: 54
NUTRIENTS PER SERVING: 102 kcal (430 kJ)

FAT ....1 g
CARBOHYDRATE..........16 g
FIBRE.............................2 g

1. Heat the oil in a saucepan, add the potato and onion and cook over medium heat for 5 minutes.

2. Add the tomato juice, wine and stock, and simmer, covered, for about 20 minutes, or until the potato is soft.

3. Add the basil leaves and purée the soup in a food processor or blender. Return to the saucepan, add salt and pepper to taste and reheat.

SERVES 8

5 ml (1 teaspoon) oil

2 medium orange sweet potatoes (about 750 g/1½ lb), peeled and chopped

1 large onion (150 g/5½ oz), coarsely chopped

500 ml (18 fl oz) tomato juice

250 ml (9 fl oz) dry white wine

500 ml (18 fl oz) prepared chicken stock

1 bunch fresh basil

salt

freshly ground black pepper

LENTIL SOUP

*A very tasty winter soup, filling and warming —
makes a meal in itself.*

•

G.I. FACTOR: 30
NUTRIENTS PER SERVING: 181 kcal (760 kJ) (serving 6)

FAT ....5 g
CARBOHYDRATE..........25 g
FIBRE...........................5 g

15 ml (1 tablespoon) oil

*1 large onion (150 g/5½ oz),
finely chopped*

*2 cloves garlic, crushed, or 2
teaspoons minced garlic*

½ teaspoon turmeric

2 teaspoons curry powder

½ teaspoon ground cumin

1 teaspoon minced chilli

1.5 litres (2½ pt) water

*375 ml (13 fl oz) prepared
chicken stock*

200 g (7 oz) red lentils

100 g (3½ oz) pearl barley

*400 g (14 oz) can tomatoes,
undrained and mashed*

salt

freshly ground black pepper

*chopped fresh parsley or
coriander, to serve*

1. Heat the oil in a large saucepan. Add the onion, cover and cook gently for about 10 minutes or until beginning to brown, stirring frequently.

2. Add the garlic, turmeric, curry powder, cumin and chilli, and cook, stirring, for 1 minute.

3. Stir in the water, stock, lentils, barley, tomatoes, and salt and pepper to taste. Bring to the boil, cover and simmer about 45 minutes or until the lentils and barley are tender.

4. Serve sprinkled with parsley or coriander.

SERVES 4 TO 6

MINESTRONE

A delicious soup that is a meal in itself.
Serve with bread and a green salad.

•

G.I. FACTOR: 37
NUTRIENTS PER SERVING: 121 kcal (510 kJ)

FAT	2 g
CARBOHYDRATE	18 g
FIBRE	7 g

1. If using dried haricot beans, soak overnight in water to cover by 5 cm (2 inches).

2. Heat a little oil in a large heavy-based saucepan. Add the onions and garlic and cook for about 5 minutes or until soft. Add the bacon bones, water, stock cubes and drained beans (soaked or canned). Bring to the boil and simmer, covered, about 2½ hours or until beans are tender. (Omit the simmering if using canned beans and simply bring to the boil.)

3. Add the carrots, celery, courgettes and tomatoes to the stock. Reduce heat and simmer, covered, for 1 hour.

4. Remove the lid, take out the bacon bones and add the macaroni to the saucepan. Continue to simmer for about 10 to 15 minutes or until the macaroni is tender.

5. Stir in the parsley and add pepper to taste. Serve with Parmesan cheese, if desired.

SERVES 6

100 g (3½ oz) dried haricot beans, or 310 g (10 oz) can, rinsed and drained

2 medium onions (240 g/8½ oz), chopped

2 cloves garlic, crushed, or 2 teaspoons minced garlic

2 bacon bones (about 300 g/ 10½ oz)

2.5 litres (4 ½ pt) water

5 beef stock cubes

3 carrots (360 g/12½ oz), diced

2 sticks celery (160 g/5½ oz), sliced

2 small courgettes (200 g/7 oz), chopped

4 tomatoes (400 g/14 oz), diced

60 g (2 oz) small macaroni

2 tablespoons chopped fresh parsley

freshly ground black pepper

grated Parmesan cheese, to serve (optional)

SPLIT PEA SOUP

A full flavoured favourite that makes an excellent basis for a light meal.
Begin this soup a day ahead, allowing the split peas to soak overnight.

•

G.I. FACTOR: 30
NUTRIENTS PER SERVING: 262 kcal (1100 kJ)

FAT	3 g
CARBOHYDRATE	39 g
FIBRE	9 g

500 g (18 oz) split peas

1 ham bone or 500 g (18 oz) bacon bones

3 litres (5pt) water

5 ml (1 teaspoon) oil

1 medium onion (120 g/4½ oz), finely chopped

1 medium carrot (120 g/4½ oz), finely chopped

1 stick celery (80 g/3 oz), finely chopped

1 bay leaf

½ teaspoon dried thyme leaves

juice of ½ lemon

freshly ground black pepper

1. Wash the split peas, place in a large saucepan with the ham bone or bacon bones and water. Bring to the boil. Allow to cool, refrigerate overnight.

2. Next day, skim any fat from the top. Bring to the boil and simmer, covered, for 2 hours.

3. Remove the bones from the soup and trim any meat from them. Return the meat to the soup.

4. Heat the oil in a frying pan, add the onion, carrot and celery and cook for about 10 minutes or until lightly browned. Add the onion mixture to the soup with the bay leaf and thyme. Simmer, covered, for 20 minutes. Remove the bay leaf.

5. Purée the soup in a food processor or blender, adding extra water if necessary to make a soup consistency.

6. Add the lemon juice and season to taste with pepper. Reheat if needed before serving.

SERVES 6

MUSHROOM AND CRACKED WHEAT SALAD

A super high fibre salad which is a variation on tabbouli. Choose small mushrooms to blend into the salad nicely.

•

G.I. FACTOR: 48

NUTRIENTS PER SERVING: 145 kcal (610 kJ)

FAT	1 g
CARBOHYDRATE	28 g
FIBRE	9 g

1. Place the burghul in a bowl and cover with cold water. Let stand for several hours or overnight.

2. Drain the burghul and squeeze out any excess water. Combine with the remaining ingredients in a bowl. Toss well and serve.

SERVES 4

160 g (5½ oz) cracked wheat (burghul)

125 g/4½ oz) button mushrooms, sliced

3 spring onions, finely chopped

25 g (1 oz) finely chopped fresh parsley

30 ml (2 tablespoons) low-oil French dressing

PASTA AND BEAN SALAD

A summer salad full of flavour.
Easy to prepare with canned beans.

•

G.I. FACTOR: 37
NUTRIENTS PER SERVING: 129 kcal (540 kJ)

FAT ....5 g
CARBOHYDRATE..........15 g
FIBRE...........................4 g

150 g (5½ oz) cooked pasta
(e.g. shells, twists)

200 g (7 oz) cooked or canned red
kidney beans, well drained

3 spring onions, finely chopped

1 tablespoon finely chopped
fresh parsley

DRESSING
15 ml (1 tablespoon) olive oil

15 ml (1 tablespoon) wine
vinegar

1 teaspoon Dijon mustard

1 clove garlic, crushed

freshly ground black pepper

1. Combine the pasta, beans, spring onions
   and parsley in a serving bowl.

2. For the dressing, combine the oil,
   vinegar, mustard, garlic and pepper in a
   screw-top jar; shake well to combine.

3. Pour the dressing over the pasta mixture
   and toss well.

SERVES 4

RED BEAN SALAD

*Serve this delicious salad over crisp
lettuce leaves if desired.*

•

G.I. FACTOR: 27
NUTRIENTS PER SERVING: 119 kcal (500 kJ)

FAT	4 g
CARBOHYDRATE	13 g
FIBRE	7 g

1. Combine the beans, onion and green pepper in a bowl.

2. For the dressing, combine all the ingredients in a screw-top jar; shake well.

3. Add the dressing to the bean mixture and toss well. Cover and refrigerate overnight to develop flavour.

SERVES 4

420 g (15 oz) can red kidney beans, rinsed and drained

1 medium white onion (120 g/4½ oz), finely chopped

1 medium green pepper (150 g/ 5½ oz), finely chopped

DRESSING

15 ml (1 tablespoon)red wine vinegar

15 ml (1 tablespoon) olive oil

pinch salt

1 teaspoon French mustard

1 clove garlic, crushed, or 1 teaspoon minced garlic

dash Tabasco sauce

freshly ground black pepper

ITALIAN BEAN SALAD

A delicious preparation which adds a new dimension to salads.

•

G.I. FACTOR: 40
NUTRIENTS PER SERVING: 270 kcal (1120 kJ)

FAT ....9 g
CARBOHYDRATE..........17 g
FIBRE...........:...............9 g

175 g (6 oz) haricot beans,
  soaked overnight in plenty of
  cold water
1 carrot, washed and cut into
  chunks
1 onion, peeled and cut in half
1 bay leaf
1 sprig of thyme
200 g (7 oz) tuna canned in brine
  or water
1 large red onion, thinly sliced
2 tablespoons chopped fresh
  parsley
salad leaves, to serve

DRESSING
½ teaspoon salt
1 large clove garlic, crushed
1 teaspoon whole grain mustard
30 ml (2 tablespoons) lemon
  juice
zest of ½ lemon
15 ml (1 tablespoon) balsamic
  vinegar
30 ml (2 tablespoons) olive oil
freshly ground black pepper

1. Discard the water that the beans were soaked in, and place the beans in a large pan with cold water to cover by 5 cm (2 inches). Add the carrot, onion and herbs, and bring to the boil, then simmer for about 1 hour or until the beans are tender.

2. Meanwhile, make the dressing by placing all the ingredients in a screw-top jar and shaking well to combine.

3. When the beans are cooked, drain them thoroughly in a colander. Remove the onion, carrot and herbs, and tip the beans into a large salad bowl. Pour the dressing over the beans while they are still warm so that the flavour permeates them.

4. Drain the tuna and break it up lightly with a fork. When the beans have cooled, add the onion rings, tuna flakes and parsley, and mix well.

5. Serve on a bed of crisp green leaves with a mixed grain roll.

SERVES 4

N.B. Italian haricot beans, known as fagioli or cannellini, work best for this dish as they have a superior flavour.

PASTA AND LENTIL SALAD

A simple, easy to prepare, filling salad dish.

•

G.I. FACTOR: 44
NUTRIENTS PER SERVING: 300 kcal (1280 kJ)

FAT	9 g
CARBOHYDRATE	43 g
FIBRE	7 g

1. Cook the pasta shapes in plenty of boiling water until just tender (al dente). Drain and, while still warm, combine with the lentils, celery, raisins and coriander.

2. To make the dressing combine all the ingredients in a screw-top jar and shake well, pour over the salad and mix well. Serve with crisp salad leaves and some thinly sliced tomato.

SERVES 4

100 g (3½ oz) dried pasta shapes

100 g (3½ oz) green lentils, soaked overnight and cooked as directed on the packet

2 large sticks celery, thinly sliced

85 g (3 oz) raisins

1 tablespoon chopped fresh coriander

salad leaves and thinly sliced tomato, to serve

DRESSING

½ teaspoon salt

3 cloves garlic, crushed

1 teaspoon mustard powder

45 ml (3 tablespoons) lemon juice

15 ml (1 tablespoon) walnut oil

15 ml (1 tablespoon) olive oil

salt and black pepper

This salad is best prepared in advance to allow the flavours to permeate the pasta.

TABBOULI

Tabbouli is best if you make it ahead, allowing time for the flavours to develop. It keeps well in the refrigerator.

•

G.I. FACTOR: 48
NUTRIENTS PER SERVING: 162 kcal (680 kJ)

FAT	10 g
CARBOHYDRATE	15 g
FIBRE	5 g

110 g (4 oz) cracked wheat (burghul)

250 ml (9 fl oz) water

50 g (2 oz) finely chopped fresh flat-leaf parsley

1 small onion (100 g/3½ oz), finely chopped

1 medium tomato (100 g/3½ oz), finely chopped

DRESSING

30 ml (2 tablespoons) fresh lemon juice

30 ml (2 tablespoons) olive oil

pinch salt

½ teaspoon freshly ground black pepper

1. Soak the burghul in the water for 1 hour, or longer if a softer texture is preferred. Drain well and squeeze out excess water.

2. Combine the burghul, parsley, onion and tomato in a bowl.

3. For the dressing, combine all the ingredients in a screw-top jar; shake well.

4. Add the dressing to the burghul mixture and toss lightly to combine.

SERVES 4

Variations include the addition of a chopped cucumber, a crushed clove of garlic or 2 tablespoons of chopped fresh mint. You can use half lemon juice and half vinegar if preferred.

BACON, BEANS AND PASTA IN TOMATO SAUCE

Top with a light sprinkling of Parmesan cheese and serve with a tossed salad.

•

G.I. FACTOR: 37
NUTRIENTS PER SERVING: 314 kcal (1320 kJ)

FAT	3 g
CARBOHYDRATE	53 g
FIBRE	12 g

1. Purée one-quarter of the beans in a food processor until very smooth. Set aside.

2. Sauté the bacon and onion in a nonstick frying pan over medium heat for about 5 to 8 minutes or until the onion is soft. Add the garlic and cook for 1 minute.

3. Add the tomatoes, tomato paste, dried herbs, stock, whole beans and puréed beans and simmer, uncovered, for about 15 to 20 minutes or until thickened to a good coating consistency.

4. Meanwhile, add the pasta to a large saucepan of boiling water, and boil, uncovered, until just tender; drain.

5. Stir the parsley into the sauce, season to taste with pepper. Toss the sauce through the drained pasta.

SERVES 6

310 g (10½ oz) can kidney beans or borlotti beans, drained

5 rashers bacon (200 g/7 oz), fat removed and chopped

1 medium onion (120 g/4½ oz), finely chopped

2 cloves garlic, crushed, or 2 teaspoons minced garlic

2 x 400 g (14 oz) can tomatoes, undrained and mashed

2 tablespoons tomato paste

1 teaspoon dried oregano leaves

1 teaspoon dried thyme leaves

250 ml (9 fl oz) prepared chicken stock

300 g (10½ oz) bow-tie pasta

15 g (½ oz) chopped fresh parsley

freshly ground black pepper

VEGETABLE LASAGNE

*A tasty, moist lasagne packed with goodies
from beans to pasta.*

•

G.I. FACTOR: 45
NUTRIENTS PER SERVING: 338 kcal (1420 kJ)

FAT	10 g
CARBOHYDRATE	44 g
FIBRE	9 g

1 bunch spinach, washed and
stalks removed

200 g (7 oz) packet instant
lasagne sheets

2 tablespoons (20 g/¼ oz) grated
Parmesan cheese or low-fat
cheddar cheese

VEGETABLE SAUCE

2 teaspoons oil

2 medium onions (240 g/9 oz),
chopped

2 cloves garlic, crushed, or
2 teaspoons minced garlic

250 g (9 oz) mushrooms, sliced

1 small green pepper (100 g/
3½ oz), chopped

140 g (5 oz) tomato paste

420 g (15 oz) can mixed beans,
rinsed and drained

420 g (15 oz) can tomatoes,
undrained and mashed

1 teaspoon dried mixed herbs

1. Blanch or lightly steam the spinach until
    just wilted; drain well.

2. For the vegetable sauce, heat the oil in a
    nonstick frying pan. Add the onions and
    garlic and cook for about 5 minutes or
    until soft. Add the mushrooms and
    green pepper and cook for a further 3
    minutes, stirring occasionally. Add the
    tomato paste, beans, tomatoes and
    herbs. Bring to the boil and simmer,
    partly covered, for 15 to 20 minutes.

3. Meanwhile, for the cheese sauce, melt
    the butter or margarine in a saucepan or
    microwave bowl. Stir in the flour and
    cook for 1 minute, stirring (for 30
    seconds 100% power, in microwave).
    Remove from the heat. Gradually add
    the milk, stirring until smooth. Stir over
    medium heat until the sauce boils and
    thickens, or in microwave (100% power)
    until boiling, stirring occasionally.
    Remove from the heat, stir in the cheese,
    nutmeg and pepper.

4. To assemble, pour half the vegetable sauce over the base of a lasagne dish, rectangular roasting tin or ovenproof dish (about 16 x 28 cm (6 x 11 inches)). Cover with a layer of lasagne sheets, then half the spinach. Spread a thin layer of cheese sauce over the spinach. Top with the remaining vegetable sauce and remaining spinach. Cover with a layer of lasagne sheets and finish with the remaining cheese sauce. Sprinkle with Parmesan or cheddar cheese.

5. Cover with aluminium foil and bake in a moderate oven (180°C/350°F/Gas Mark 4) for 40 minutes. Remove foil and bake for a further 30 minutes or until the top is beginning to brown.

SERVES 6

CHEESE SAUCE

20 g (¾ oz) butter or margarine

1 tablespoon plain flour

375 ml (13 fl oz) semi-skimmed milk

60 g (2 oz) grated low-fat cheese

pinch ground nutmeg

freshly ground black pepper

TIP

Dipping the lasagne sheets briefly in hot water before use helps to soften them prior to cooking.

CREAMY MUSHROOMS AND PASTA

When mushrooms are plentiful put this dish together quickly with ingredients from the pantry.

•

G.I. FACTOR: 41

NUTRIENTS PER SERVING: 443 kcal (1860 kJ)

FAT	7 g
CARBOHYDRATE	68 g
FIBRE	8 g

300 g 10½ oz) macaroni or other small pasta

2 tablespoons finely chopped fresh parsley

2 tablespoons (20 g/¼ oz) finely grated Parmesan cheese

SAUCE

10 ml (2 teaspoons) olive oil

1 medium onion (120 g/4½ oz), finely sliced

1 clove garlic, crushed, or 1 teaspoon minced garlic

500 g (18 oz) mushrooms

1 teaspoon paprika

2 teaspoons Dijon mustard

2 tablespoons tomato paste

375 ml (13 fl oz) can evaporated skimmed milk

30 g (1 oz) grated low-fat cheddar cheese

40 g (1½ oz) chopped spring onions

freshly ground black pepper

1. Add the pasta to a large saucepan of boiling water, and boil, uncovered, until just tender; drain and keep warm.

2. While the pasta is cooking, begin the sauce. Heat the oil in a nonstick frying pan. Add the onion, garlic and mushrooms, and cook for about 5 minutes or until softened.

3. Combine the paprika, mustard, tomato paste and milk in a small jug. Stir into the mushroom mixture with the cheese, and cook, stirring frequently, over low heat for 5 minutes.

4. Add the spring onions with pepper to taste.

5. Pour the sauce over the pasta and toss gently to combine. Serve sprinkled with the parsley and Parmesan cheese.

SERVES 4

Mushrooms are a good source of niacin and can be a source of Vitamin B12 if they are grown on a mixture containing animal compost.

Carnation Lite™ evaporated skimmed milk is available in 215 g cartons from leading supermarkets.

FETTUCCINE WITH BACON AND MUSHROOM SAUCE

This is a tasty, low-fat variation on the traditional creamy sauce of this popular pasta dish. Serve with a tossed green salad.

•

G.I. FACTOR: 41
NUTRIENTS PER SERVING: 359 kcal (1510 kJ)

FAT	10 g
CARBOHYDRATE	47 g
FIBRE	4 g

1. Cut the bacon into short, thin slices. Cook in a nonstick frying pan until browned. Meanwhile, add the fettuccine to a large saucepan of boiling water, and boil, uncovered, until just tender; drain.

2. Add the mushrooms and oil to the frying pan, cook for 2 minutes.

3. Stir in the mustard and wine and cook for a further 3 minutes. Reduce the heat, add the cheese and stir until melted.

4. Add the blended cornflour and water, stir over low heat until the mixture becomes quite thick.

5. Remove from the heat and cool slightly. Gradually add the buttermilk and pepper, stirring until well combined. Do not heat or the sauce may curdle.

6. Serve the sauce immediately over the fettuccine. Serve with Parmesan cheese, if desired.

SERVES 4

4 rashers (about 160 g/5½ oz) bacon, fat removed

250 g (9 oz) fettuccine pasta

70 g (2½ oz) small mushrooms, sliced

15 ml (1 tablespoon) oil

1 teaspoon wholegrain mustard

30 ml (2 tablespoons) red or white wine (optional)

30 g (1 oz) grated low-fat cheddar cheese

2 teaspoons cornflour blended with 30 ml (2 tablespoons) water

125 ml (4½ fl oz) buttermilk

freshly ground black pepper

grated Parmesan cheese, to serve (optional)

MAINS AND ACCOMPANIMENTS

CHICKEN AND BASMATI RICE PILAU

CREAMY VEGETABLE AND CHICK PEA CURRY

CURRY RICE WITH CHICKEN SAUCE

CHILLI BEAN RISOTTO

VEAL, VEGETABLE AND PASTA STIR-FRY

BEEF AND LENTIL RISSOLES

SPAGHETTI BOLOGNESE

MEGA-VEG MEAT LOAF

FISH WITH SPICY BEANS AND TOMATO

PARSLEY CHEESE PIE

ROASTED VEGETABLE AND PASTA BAKE

WINTER CHILLI HOTPOT

FRIED BASMATI RICE

A SIDE DISH OF LENTILS

MIXED BEAN ACCOMPANIMENT

SPICY NOODLES

SUMMER BARLEY

SWEET POTATO AND CORN FRITTERS

●

CHICKEN AND BASMATI RICE PILAU

This is a flavoursome one-pot meal, best served with a salad.

•

G.I. FACTOR: 59
NUTRIENTS PER SERVING: 614 kcal (2580 kJ)

FAT..............................13 g
CARBOHYDRATE..........84 g
FIBRE............................3 g

1. Heat the oil in a medium to large saucepan, add the chicken and cook, stirring, over medium heat for about 10 minutes or until beginning to brown. Transfer to a plate.

2. Melt the butter in the same pan, add the onion and red pepper, and cook for about 5 minutes or until soft.

3. Add the rosemary and cook for a further 3 minutes or until the onion is lightly browned. Return the chicken to the pan, add the rice and stir.

4. Pour the cold stock over the chicken and rice mixture and bring to the boil. Cover with a tight-fitting lid and simmer gently for 20 minutes or until the rice is tender and the liquid is absorbed.

SERVES 2 AS A MAIN COURSE

5 ml (1 teaspoon) olive oil

2 chicken thigh fillets (about 250 g/9 oz), skinned and sliced

10 g (½ oz) butter

1 large (150 g/5½ oz) purple Spanish onion, sliced

½ medium red pepper (75 g/2½ oz), sliced

½ teaspoon dried rosemary leaves

200 g (7 oz) Basmati rice

500 ml (18 fl oz) prepared chicken stock

This uses chicken thigh fillets which should be well trimmed to remove all visible fat. Being rice-based, the dish is very high in carbohydrate and good for active people.

CREAMY VEGETABLE AND CHICK PEA CURRY

This curry is high in protein and iron thanks to the addition of chick peas. Cut the pumpkin into 3 cm (1½ inch) cubes before weighing.

•

G.I. FACTOR: 44
NUTRIENTS PER SERVING: 210 kcal (880 kJ)

FAT	6 g
CARBOHYDRATE	30 g
FIBRE	8 g

150 g (5½ oz) dried chick peas, soaked overnight

5 ml (1 teaspoon) oil

1 medium onion (120 g/4 oz), chopped

2 cloves garlic, crushed, or 2 teaspoons minced garlic

1 tablespoon minced ginger

2 teaspoons ground cumin

2 teaspoons ground coriander

2 teaspoons turmeric

2 teaspoons curry powder

½ teaspoon minced chilli

250 ml (9 fl oz) chicken stock

1 large potato (120 g/4 oz), cut into 3 cm (1½ inch) cubes

240 g (8½ oz) cubed pumpkin

2 carrots (240 g/8½ oz), thickly sliced

400 g (14 oz) can tomatoes, undrained and chopped

1. Drain the chick peas, place in a large saucepan. Add fresh water to cover by 5 cm (2 inches) and bring to the boil. Simmer, covered, for 1 hour over a low heat. Drain and set aside.

2. Heat the oil in the saucepan, add the onion, garlic and ginger and cook for about 5 minutes or until the onion is soft. Add the spices and chilli, then cook for a further 2 minutes. Add the stock, potato, pumpkin, carrots, tomatoes and chick peas, cover, and simmer for 20 minutes.

3. Add the red pepper and courgettes and simmer for a further 10 minutes.

4. Meanwhile, for the creamy chicken sauce, melt the butter or margarine in a small saucepan. Add the flour and cook for 2 minutes, stirring constantly. Remove from the heat and gradually stir in the stock. Stir over heat until the sauce boils and thickens.

5. Remove from the heat and gradually whisk in the evaporated milk until blended.

6. Add the creamy chicken sauce to the curried vegetables and mix gently. Allow to heat through, then serve immediately.

    SERVES 6

1 large red pepper (150 g/5½ oz), thickly sliced

4 small courgettes (400 g/14 oz), thickly sliced

CREAMY CHICKEN SAUCE

20 g (¾ oz) butter or margarine

1 tablespoon plain flour

250 ml (9 fl oz) prepared chicken stock

125 ml (4½ fl oz) evaporated skimmed milk

CURRY RICE WITH CHICKEN SAUCE

This is a very high carbohydrate dish and a good choice for all sports people.

•

G.I. FACTOR: 58

NUTRIENTS PER SERVING: 483 kcal (2030 kJ)

FAT............................10 g
CARBOHYDRATE..........64 g
FIBRE...........................3 g

2 boned chicken breasts (about 375 g/13 oz), skin removed

15 ml (1 tablespoon) oil

1 large onion (150 g/5½ oz), finely chopped

1 stick celery (80 g/3 oz), sliced

1 medium carrot (120 g/4 oz), grated

6 sprigs fresh parsley, finely chopped

125 ml (4½ fl oz) dry white wine

2 teaspoons tomato paste

125 ml (4½ fl oz) prepared chicken stock

freshly ground black pepper

1 bay leaf

2 tablespoons (20 g/¾ oz) grated Parmesan cheese, to serve

RICE

750 ml (1¼ pt) water

300 g (10½ oz) Basmati rice

5 g (¼ oz) butter or margarine

1 teaspoon curry powder

1. Cut the chicken into 1 cm (½ inch) cubes.

2. Heat the oil in a saucepan or nonstick frying pan. Add the vegetables and parsley, and cook gently for 10 minutes, stirring frequently.

3. Add the chicken and cook, stirring, for 4 to 5 minutes. Add the wine and boil quickly until it evaporates. Stir in the combined tomato paste and stock. Season with pepper and add the bay leaf. Bring to the boil, reduce the heat and simmer gently for 15 minutes. Remove the bay leaf.

4. Meanwhile, cook the rice. Bring the water to the boil in a saucepan, add the rice and simmer, covered, for about 18 to 20 minutes or until all the water is absorbed. Drain and rinse well under hot water. Return to the saucepan, add the butter or margarine and curry powder, stir until combined.

5. Place the rice in a warmed serving dish, top with the chicken sauce and sprinkle with the Parmesan cheese.

SERVES 4

CHILLI BEAN RISOTTO

This tasty and different risotto should be served with a crisp salad..

•

G.I. FACTOR: 58

NUTRIENTS PER SERVING: 450 kcal (1880 kJ)

FAT ....6 g
CARBOHYDRATE..........55 g
FIBRE............................6 g

1. If using dried beans, rinse them well with cold water and then place them in a saucepan, cover with fresh water and bring to the boil. Boil for 1 minute, then turn off the heat and leave to soak for 2 hours. After 2 hours, pour off the water and cover with fresh cold water. Bring to the boil and boil gently for 1½ to 2 hours, or until the beans are tender. Drain well. Canned beans simply need draining and rinsing before use.

2. To make the risotto, heat the oil in a large frying pan and fry the bacon, onion and garlic until golden.

3. Drain the sun-dried tomatoes and roughly chop. Add the rice to the pan and stir well to coat it with oil.

4. Mix the tomato paste with the stock and pour into the pan. Stir in the cayenne and paprika and add the courgette, pepper, tomatoes and beans.

5. Bring to a simmer, cover the pan and simmer gently for 15 minutes or until the rice is tender, adding a little more water if necessary.
   SERVES 4 (large portions); can stretch to 6

If you prefer your food less spicy, substitute mild paprika for hot paprika.

100 g (3½ oz) dried, or 1 small can red kidney beans (about 200 g/7 oz)

15 ml (1 tablespoon) olive oil

85 g (3 oz) lean smoked bacon, trimmed of visible fat and chopped

1 large red onion (150 g/5½ oz), chopped

2 cloves garlic, crushed, or 2 teaspoons minced garlic

50 g (2 oz) sun-dried tomatoes (these should be purchased dry and not soaked in oil, and need to be covered with boiling water and soaked for 30 minutes)

200 g (7 oz) Basmati rice

1 heaped tablespoon tomato paste

600 ml (1 pt) prepared chicken stock

good pinch cayenne pepper

1 heaped tablespoon hot paprika

1 medium courgette, roughly chopped

1 medium pepper, sliced

VEAL, VEGETABLE AND PASTA STIR-FRY

*Loaded with vegetables, this high carbohydrate dish
is a very low-fat main meal.*

•

G.I. FACTOR: 44
NUTRIENTS PER SERVING: 340 kcal (1430 kJ)

FAT ....3 g
CARBOHYDRATE..........54 g
FIBRE ....10 g

400 g (14 oz) spaghetti
10 ml (2 teaspoons) oil
1 medium onion (120 g/4 oz),
   chopped
1 tablespoon grated fresh ginger
   or 1 tablespoon minced ginger
1 clove garlic, crushed, or
   1 teaspoon minced garlic
200 g (7 oz) veal steaks, cut into
   thin strips
1 stick celery (80 g/3 oz), sliced
1 small yellow pepper (100 g/3½
   oz), chopped
1 medium red pepper (150 g/5½
   oz), chopped
200 g (7 oz) cauliflower, cut into
   florets
1 large carrot (150 g/5½ oz),
   chopped
200 g (7 oz) broccoli, chopped
350 g (12 oz) flat mushrooms,
   sliced
1 bunch fresh asparagus, chopped
15 ml (1 tablespoon) salt-reduced
   soy sauce
60 ml (2 fl oz) black bean sauce
1½ tablespoons cornflour
165 ml (6 fl oz) water

1. Add the spaghetti to a large saucepan of boiling water, and boil, uncovered, until just tender; drain and keep warm.

2. Heat the oil in a wok or large nonstick frying pan. Add the onion, ginger, garlic and veal. Stir-fry over medium heat for about 3 to 5 minutes or until the veal is almost cooked.

3. Add the remaining vegetables and stir-fry until just tender, sprinkling in a little water if necessary.

4. Blend together the sauces, cornflour and water. Stir into the vegetables until the mixture boils and thickens.

5. Add the spaghetti; stir until heated through. Serve immediately.

SERVES 6

Almost any selection of colourful vegetables can be used.

BEEF AND LENTIL RISSOLES

*Serve these succulent rissoles hot with vegetables or
salad and mustard or chutney.*

•

G.I. FACTOR: 34
NUTRIENTS PER RISSOLE: 74 kcal (310 kJ)

FAT	3 g
CARBOHYDRATE	6 g
FIBRE	7 g

1. Cook the lentils in a saucepan of boiling water for about 20 minutes or until soft; drain well.

2. Combine the lentils with the beef, onion, pepper, garlic, herbs, ketchup, egg and black pepper in a bowl; mix well.

3. Add enough oat bran to form a burger consistency. Shape the mixture into 24 rissoles and place on a lightly greased baking tray.

4. Bake in a hot oven (200°C/400°F/Gas Mark 6) for about 40 minutes, or until cooked through, turning halfway through cooking time. Alternatively, cook the rissoles in a nonstick frying pan over medium-high heat or until browned and cooked through.

MAKES 24 SMALL RISSOLES

100 g (3½ oz) red lentils

400 g (14 oz) lean minced beef

1 medium onion (120 g/4 oz), finely chopped

½ small pepper (50 g/2 oz), finely chopped

1 clove garlic, crushed, or 1 teaspoon minced garlic

2 teaspoons dried mixed herbs

80 ml (3 fl oz) tomato ketchup

1 egg, lightly beaten

freshly ground black pepper

about 70 g (2½ oz) unprocessed oat bran

Reheat the leftovers and serve sandwiched in Lebanese pitta bread with chutney, tomato, cucumber, grated carrot and lettuce.

SPAGHETTI BOLOGNESE

*To keep the fat content down, use a minimum amount of oil
and the leanest possible minced beef.*

•

G.I. FACTOR: 43
NUTRIENTS PER SERVING: 545 kcal (2290 kJ)

FAT	14 g
CARBOHYDRATE	72 g
FIBRE	7 g

15 ml (1 tablespoon) olive oil

1 very small onion (80 g/3 oz),
  finely chopped

1 carrot (100 g/3½ oz), grated

1 stick celery (80 g/3 oz), sliced

1 rasher (40 g/1½ oz) bacon, fat
  removed, finely chopped

2 cloves garlic, crushed, or
  2 teaspoons minced garlic

300 g (10½ oz) lean minced beef

2 tablespoons tomato paste

400 g (14 oz) can tomatoes,
  undrained and mashed

60 ml (2 fl oz) dry red wine

60 ml (2 fl oz) beef stock

¼ teaspoon dried oregano leaves

freshly ground black pepper

1 bay leaf

2 pinches grated nutmeg

375 g (13 oz) spaghetti

chopped fresh parsley, to serve
  (optional)

grated Parmesan cheese

1. Heat the oil in a saucepan or frying pan,
   add the onion, carrot, celery, bacon and
   garlic and cook for about 10 minutes, or
   until the onion is very soft, stirring
   frequently. Cover if drying out too
   much.

2. Increase the heat and add the beef. Cook
   for about 5 minutes, stirring constantly
   until the beef is crumbly and browned.

3. Add the tomato paste, tomatoes, wine
   and stock. Bring to the boil. Add the
   oregano, pepper, bay leaf and nutmeg
   and stir thoroughly. Cover and simmer
   for 1 hour, stirring frequently to prevent
   sticking. Remove the bay leaf.

4. Meanwhile, add the spaghetti to a large
   saucepan of boiling water and boil,
   uncovered, until just tender; drain.

5. Serve the beef sauce over the spaghetti.
   Sprinkle with parsley and serve with
   Parmesan cheese, if desired.

SERVES 4

MEGA-VEG MEAT LOAF

A very moist and tender meat loaf. By adding plenty of vegetables to the meat, the fat content of the whole dish is reduced.

•

G.I. FACTOR: 62
NUTRIENTS PER SERVING: 338 kcal (1420 kJ)

FAT	12 g
CARBOHYDRATE	21 g
FIBRE	4 g

1. Heat the oil in a nonstick frying pan, add the onion, garlic and mushrooms and cook for about 5 minutes or until just soft; cool.

2. Combine the remaining ingredients in a large bowl. Add the onion mixture and mix well.

3. Press the mixture into a lightly oiled loaf tin (about 15 x 25 cm/6 x 10 inches). Cover with a lid or foil and stand in a baking dish. Pour enough hot water into the baking dish to come halfway up the sides of the loaf tin.

4. Bake in a hot oven (200°C/400°F/Gas Mark 6) for about 1 hour or until cooked through.

SERVES 6

5 ml (1 teaspoon) oil

1 medium onion (120 g/4 oz), finely chopped

1 clove garlic, crushed, or 1 teaspoon minced garlic

100 g (3½ oz) small mushrooms, finely sliced

500 g (18 oz) lean minced beef

90 g (3½ oz) rolled oats

1 small courgette (100 g/3½ oz), grated

1 medium carrot (120 g/4 oz), grated

75 g (3 oz) green peas

30 ml (2 tablespoons) tomato ketchup

5 ml (1 teaspoon) Worcestershire sauce

1 egg, lightly beaten

1 teaspoon dried basil leaves

½ teaspoon dried oregano leaves

½ teaspoon dried thyme leaves

4 tablespoons finely chopped fresh parsley

FISH WITH SPICY BEANS AND TOMATO

Serve this dish alongside Basmati rice.

•

G.I. FACTOR: 27

NUTRIENTS PER SERVING: 205 kcal (860 kJ)

FAT ....4 g
CARBOHYDRATE ....7 g
FIBRE...........................4 g

10 ml (2 teaspoons) oil

1 stick celery (80 g/3 oz), finely diced

1 medium onion (120 g/4 oz), finely chopped

1 clove garlic, crushed, or 1 teaspoon minced garlic

400 g (14 oz) can tomatoes, undrained and mashed

300 g (10½ oz) can butter beans, well drained

1 teaspoon minced chilli

125 ml (4½ fl oz) dry white wine

4 boneless white fish fillets (about 500 g/18 oz), cut into cubes

2 tablespoons chopped fresh parsley

freshly ground black pepper

1. Heat the oil in a nonstick frying pan or saucepan. Add the celery, onion and garlic and cook for about 5 minutes or until softened. Add the tomatoes, beans and chilli. Simmer, uncovered, for 10 minutes.

2. Meanwhile, heat the wine in a medium saucepan over moderate heat. Add the fish and poach gently for about 3 to 4 minutes or until just cooked through.

3. Combine the undrained fish with the tomato and bean mixture. Add the parsley with pepper to taste. Serve immediately.

SERVES 4

PARSLEY CHEESE PIE

A cheese and egg dish incorporating rice.
Serve with a tossed salad.

•

G.I. FACTOR: 51
NUTRIENTS PER SERVING: 207 kcal (870 kJ)

FAT ....8 g
CARBOHYDRATE..........19 g
FIBRE...........................3 g

1. Add the rice to a saucepan of boiling water, and boil, uncovered, for about 12 minutes or until just tender; drain.

2. Combine the rice, parsley, half the cheese, the onion, creamed corn, corn kernels, courgette and mushrooms in a bowl and spoon into a greased 25 cm (10 inch) pie dish.

3. Whisk the eggs, milk, nutmeg and cumin in a bowl. Fold in the lightly beaten egg white and pour evenly over the rice mixture. Sprinkle the remaining cheese on top.

4. Bake in a moderate oven (180°C/350°F/ Gas Mark 4) for about 1 hour or until set in the centre.

SERVES 6

100 g (3½ oz) Basmati rice

50 g (2 oz) chopped fresh parsley

125 g (4½ oz) grated low-fat cheddar cheese

1 large (150 g/5½ oz) onion, finely chopped

130 g (4½ oz) creamed corn

130 g (4½ oz) corn kernels

1 large courgette (180 g/6 oz), grated

35 g (1½ oz) mushrooms, finely chopped

3 eggs

500 ml (18 fl oz) semi-skimmed milk

¼ teaspoon grated nutmeg

1 teaspoon ground cumin

1 egg-white, lightly beaten

ROASTED VEGETABLE AND PASTA BAKE

A delicious, filling main course, best served with a salad.

•

G.I. FACTOR: 48
NUTRIENTS PER SERVING: 595 kcal (2499 kJ)

FAT..............................16 g
CARBOHYDRATE..........91 g
FIBRE ....10 g

1 head of fennel, trimmed and
  cut into wedges
1 red pepper, cut into 2 cm
  (¾ inch) squares
1 yellow pepper, cut into 2 cm
  (¾ inch) squares
2 medium courgettes, cut into
  cubes
1 small aubergine, cut into cubes
450 g (1 lb) cherry tomatoes
2 red onions, cut into chunks
2 cloves garlic, finely chopped
15 g (½ oz) fresh basil, roughly
  chopped
15 ml (1 tablespoon) olive oil
200 g (7 oz) dried pasta, such as
  penne or rigatoni
150 g (5½ oz) reduced-fat
  mozzarella cheese,cubed
1 tablespoon grated Parmesan
  cheese

SAUCE
570 ml (20 fl oz) skimmed milk
35 g (1½ oz) plain flour
25 g (1 oz) polyunsaturated
  margarine
salt and pepper
nutmeg

1. Pre-heat the oven to 240°C/475°F/Gas
    Mark 9.
2. Place all the vegetables in a large bowl,
    add the garlic, basil and oil, mix
    thoroughly and then spread in a
    roasting tin. Bake in the oven for 35
    minutes until the vegetables are roasted
    and slightly charred at the edges.
3. Meanwhile, to make the sauce, place the
    milk, flour and margarine in a saucepan
    and whisk together over a low heat until
    the sauce begins to simmer and thicken.
    Turn the heat down very low and
    simmer for a further 3 minutes. Season
    with salt and pepper and a good grating
    of nutmeg. Remove from the heat, cover
    and leave on one side. Cook the pasta in
    plenty of boiling water until just tender.
4. When the vegetables are cooked, remove
    them and turn down the oven to
    180°C/350°F/Gas Mark 4. Mix together
    the pasta, vegetables and sauce in a large
    bowl. Add the cubed mozzarella and stir
    well. Turn the mixture into a lightly
    greased ovenproof dish, cover with a lid
    or foil and bake for 40 minutes.
5. Remove the foil and sprinkle Parmesan
    cheese over the surface before serving.
    SERVES 4 (generous servings)

WINTER CHILLI HOTPOT

A tasty one-pot meal that can be prepared in around 30 minutes using canned beans. You could serve it with a crusty roll and side salad.

•

G.I. FACTOR: 38
NUTRIENTS PER SERVING: 264 kcal (1110 kJ) (serving 6)

FAT	1.5 g
CARBOHYDRATE	47 g
FIBRE	12 g

1. If using dried beans, soak overnight in water to cover by 5 cm (2 inches). Drain. Bring the 1.2 litres (2 pt) water to the boil in a large saucepan, add the beans and bay leaf. Boil rapidly for 15 minutes, then reduce heat and simmer for 40 minutes. Drain and set aside.

2. Heat the oil in a nonstick frying pan, add the onion and garlic and cook for about 5 minutes or until soft.

3. Add the celery, courgettes and mushrooms, and cook, stirring, for 5 minutes. Stir in the beans (cooked or canned), tomatoes, chilli, tomato paste and stock, and bring to the boil.

4. Add the macaroni, reduce the heat and simmer for about 20 minutes or until the pasta is tender. Add pepper to taste and serve sprinkled with parsley.

SERVES 4 TO 6

180 g (6 oz) dried red kidney beans or 420 g (15 oz) can kidney beans, rinsed and drained

1.2 litres (2 pt) water

1 bay leaf

5 ml (1 teaspoon) oil

1 onion, finely chopped

2 cloves garlic, crushed, or 2 teaspoons minced garlic

2 sticks celery (160 g/5½ oz), sliced

2 small courgettes (200 g/7 oz), sliced

250 g (9 oz) button mushrooms

2 x 400 g (28 oz) can tomatoes, undrained and chopped

1 teaspoon minced chilli

2 tablespoons tomato paste

375 ml (13 fl oz) prepared vegetable stock

250 g (9 oz) small macaroni

freshly ground black pepper

chopped fresh parsley, to serve

FRIED BASMATI RICE

Serve as a light meal or an
accompaniment to a stir-fry.

•

G.I. FACTOR: 56
NUTRIENTS PER SERVING: 443 kcal (1860 kJ) (serving 6)

FAT	14 g
CARBOHYDRATE	65 g
FIBRE	5 g

400 g (14 oz) Basmati rice

30 ml (2 tablespoons) oil

3 large eggs, lightly beaten

2 large slices gammon, chopped

1 cm (½ inch) piece fresh ginger,
   very thinly sliced, or
   1 teaspoon minced ginger

150 g (5½ oz) cooked green peas

270 g (10 oz) can corn kernels,
   drained

4 spring onions, sliced

22 ml (1½ tablespoons) oyster
   sauce

10 ml (2 teaspoons) soy sauce

15 ml (1 tablespoon) chicken
   stock

2.5 ml (½ teaspoon) sesame oil

1. Place the rice in a saucepan with enough water to cover by 2.5 cm (1 inch). Bring to the boil, cover with a tight-fitting lid and simmer very gently for 20 minutes. Remove from the heat, stir with a fork to separate the grains and set aside to cool.

2. Heat half the oil in a frying pan, add the eggs and cook over medium heat, stirring with a fork, for 2 to 3 minutes or until set. Remove from pan and cool.

3. Heat the remaining oil in the same pan and stir-fry the gammon.

4. Add the rice to the frying pan. Stir in the ginger, peas, corn and onions and toss gently until heated through. Add the sauces, stock and sesame oil and stir to coat the rice thoroughly.

5. Stir in the egg and serve immediately.

SERVES 4 TO 6
AS A LIGHT MAIN COURSE

A SIDE DISH OF LENTILS

This dish using lentils is full of flavour and is an excellent accompaniment to steak or chicken. The chilli can be adjusted to taste!

•

G.I. FACTOR: 29
NUTRIENTS PER SERVING: 71 kcal (300 kJ)

FAT	3 g
CARBOHYDRATE	7 g
FIBRE	4 g

1. Place the lentils in a saucepan with enough water to cover. Bring to the boil and boil, covered, for about 10 to 15 minutes, or until cooked but firm. Drain.

2. Heat the oil in a separate saucepan, add the onion, chillies and garlic and cook for about 5 minutes or until the onion is soft.

3. Add the lentils, tomatoes and cumin and cook until heated through. Add salt and pepper to taste.

SERVES 6 AS AN
ACCOMPANIMENT

150 g (5½ oz) dried green or brown lentils

15 ml (1 tablespoon) olive oil

1 small onion (80 g/3 oz), chopped

2 fresh small red chillies, seeded and finely chopped, or 2 teaspoons minced red chilli

1 clove garlic, crushed, or 1 teaspoon minced garlic

2 medium tomatoes (200 g/7 oz), finely chopped

1 teaspoon ground cumin

pinch salt

freshly ground black pepper

MIXED BEAN ACCOMPANIMENT

*A very refreshing salad which makes a nice
accompaniment to a main meal.*

•

G.I. FACTOR: 40

NUTRIENTS PER SERVING: 71 kcal (300 kJ)

FAT ....neg.
CARBOHYDRATE..........12 g
FIBRE ....5 g

*310 g (10½ oz) can mixed beans,
rinsed and drained*

*2 sticks celery (160 g/6 oz),
finely diced*

*1 medium pepper (150 g/5½ oz),
finely diced*

4 spring onions, finely chopped

*1 tablespoon chopped fresh
parsley*

*2 teaspoons chopped fresh mint
(optional)*

*45 ml (3 tablespoons) low-oil
French dressing*

1. Combine all the ingredients in a serving
   bowl; mix well.

2. Let stand for 1 hour before serving to
   allow the flavours to develop.

SERVES 4

SPICY NOODLES

Serve these extra-spicy noodles alongside something plain or as part of a stir-fry with vegetables.

•

G.I. FACTOR: 34
NUTRIENTS PER SERVING: 278 kcal (1170 kJ)

FAT .... 6 g
CARBOHYDRATE .... 45 g
FIBRE .... 4 g

1. Add the noodles to a large saucepan of boiling water, and boil, uncovered, for about 5 minutes or until just tender.

2. While the noodles are cooking, heat the oil in a nonstick frying pan, add the garlic, ginger, chilli and spring onions and stir-fry for 1 minute. Remove from the heat.

3. Stir in the peanut butter and soy sauce and gradually add the stock, stirring until smooth. Stir over heat until simmering, and simmer for 2 minutes.

4. Drain the noodles and add to the spicy sauce, stirring to coat. Serve immediately.

SERVES 4 AS AN
ACCOMPANIMENT

250 g (9 oz) dried thin egg noodles

10 ml (2 teaspoons) oil

2 cloves garlic, crushed, or 2 teaspoons minced garlic

1 teaspoon minced ginger

1 teaspoon minced chilli

6 spring onions, sliced

1 tablespoon smooth peanut butter

30 ml (2 tablespoons) soy sauce

250 ml (9 fl oz) prepared chicken stock

SUMMER BARLEY

*Try barley as a terrific low G.I. accompaniment to a main meal.
Prepared this way it is very tasty but does take some time to cook.*

●

G.I. FACTOR: 25
NUTRIENTS PER SERVING: 212 kcal (890 kJ)

FAT ....7 g
CARBOHYDRATE..........33 g
FIBRE...........................5 g

1 large red pepper (200 g/7 oz),
cut into strips

15 ml (1 tablespoon) olive oil

200 g (7 oz) pearl barley

750 ml (1¼ pt) prepared chicken
stock

60 g (2 oz) grated Parmesan or
low-fat cheddar cheese
(optional)

1. Toss the pepper and oil together in a
large casserole dish. Bake in a hot oven
(200°C/400°F/Gas Mark 6) for 30
minutes.

2. Add the barley and stir until coated with
oil. Add the stock, cover tightly and bake
for about 1 hour or until all the stock is
absorbed and the barley is tender — add
extra stock if necessary.

3. Do not stir the mixture once cooked.
Cover and keep warm until ready to
serve. Serve with cheese, if desired.

SERVES 4 AS AN
ACCOMPANIMENT

SWEET POTATO AND CORN FRITTERS

A different and easy way to serve potato. The sweet potato gives the fritters a distinctive flavour and lowers the GI factor.

•

G.I. FACTOR: 56
NUTRIENTS PER FRITTER: 121 kcal (510 kJ)

FAT	2 g
CARBOHYDRATE	22 g
FIBRE	3 g

1. Combine the potatoes and onion and steam or microwave together until the potatoes are tender.

2. Mash the potatoes and onion with the egg. Add the corn, pepper to taste, rolled oats and self-raising flour; mix until well combined.

3. Refrigerate the mixture for 30 minutes or until completely cooled (this makes it much easier to shape).

4. Shape the mixture into 8 rounds, coating gently with extra flour.

5. Heat the oil in a nonstick frying pan to just cover the base. Add the rounds in a single layer and cook over moderate heat, about 4 minutes each side or until browned.

MAKES 8 FRITTERS

1 medium orange sweet potato (375 g/13 oz), peeled and roughly chopped

2 new potatoes (200 g/7 oz), peeled and roughly chopped

1 medium onion (120 g/4 oz), finely chopped

1 egg, lightly beaten

270 g (10 oz) can corn kernels

freshly ground black pepper

45 g (1½ oz) rolled oats

2 tablespoons self-raising flour

extra flour

5 ml (1 teaspoon) oil

New potatoes do not mash easily but are used here because they tend to have lower G.I.s than other potatoes.

DESSERTS

APPLE CUSTARD CRISP

APPLE SHELL PUDDING

BAKED APPLES

CREAMED RICE WITH SLICED PEARS

CREAMY APRICOT SLICE

REFRESHING FRUIT CHEESECAKE

YOGHURT BERRY JELLY

FRUIT COMPOTE

•

APPLE CUSTARD CRISP

•

G.I. FACTOR: 52
NUTRIENTS PER SERVING: 269 kcal (1130 kJ) (serving 6)

FAT..............................10 g
CARBOHYDRATE..........42 g
FIBRE............................4 g

1. Peel and core the apples and cut into thin slices. Drizzle with lemon juice. Microwave (100% power) for 5 to 8 minutes, or lightly stew in a saucepan, until just tender.

2. Add the apricots and raisins. Place in a well-greased ovenproof dish.

3. Blend the custard powder and sugar with a little of the milk in a small saucepan or microwave jug. Add the remaining milk and heat gently, or microwave (100% power), until the custard boils and thickens. Pour over the apple mixture.

4. Melt the butter and honey in a small saucepan or in the microwave. Combine with the rolled oats, flour, spices and nuts. Sprinkle over the apple and custard mixture.

5. Bake in a moderate oven (180°C/350°F/ Gas Mark 4) for about 30 minutes or until the topping is browned.

SERVES 4 TO 6

4 medium to large Granny Smith apples (about 650 g/1¼ lb)

juice of 1 lemon

8 dried apricot halves, chopped

40 g (1½ oz) raisins or sultanas

1 tablespoon custard powder

2 teaspoons sugar

185 ml (6 fl oz) semi-skimmed milk

40 g (1½ oz) butter

22 ml (1½ tablespoons) honey

90 g (3½ oz) rolled oats

55 g (2 oz) plain flour, sifted

1 teaspoon ground cinnamon

½ teaspoon ground allspice

1 tablespoon chopped walnuts or pecans

APPLE SHELL PUDDING

A different way to eat pasta and a good way to use up leftover cooked pasta. Serve this accompanied by a low-fat custard or fresh fruit salad.

•

G.I. FACTOR: 41

NUTRIENTS PER SERVING: 207 kcal (870 kJ)

FAT ....4 g
CARBOHYDRATE..........39 g
FIBRE...........................2 g

2 eggs

450 g (1 lb) cooked small
  pasta shells

110 g (4 oz) sugar

1 teaspoon ground cinnamon

½ teaspoon mixed spice

300 g (10½ oz) grated apple

15 g (½ oz) butter or margarine,
  melted

1. Whisk the eggs in a bowl until thick, add all the remaining ingredients. Stir until well combined.

2. Pour the mixture into a greased shallow baking dish. Bake in a moderate oven (180°C/350°F/Gas Mark 4) for about 40 minutes or until set in the centre.

SERVES 6

You will need to cook 270 g (9½ oz) pasta.

BAKED APPLES

*Tender cooked apples, stuffed with plump dried fruits
make an easy low G.I. dessert.*

•

G.I. FACTOR: 45
NUTRIENTS PER SERVING: 243 kcal (1020 kJ)

FAT .... 4 g
CARBOHYDRATE .... 52 g
FIBRE .... 4 g

1. Core the apples, keeping them whole. Remove the peel from around one end and in strips around each apple (to give a striped appearance).

2. Combine the currants, sultanas, prunes, apricots, lemon zest, cinnamon and jam in a small bowl. Stuff the mixture into the apple centres.

3. Place the apples in a baking dish just large enough to hold them.

4. Combine the butter, honey, orange juice and nutmeg in a small saucepan. Stir over low heat until the butter is melted. Pour over the apples. Bake in a moderate oven (180°C/350°F/Gas Mark 4) for about 40 minutes, or until the apples are tender but not mushy, basting with the juices every 10 minutes.

5. Serve the apples drizzled with some of the juices from the dish.

SERVES 4

4 large Golden Delicious apples (800 g/1¼ lb)

15 g (½ oz) currants

15 g (½ oz) sultanas

4 prunes, pitted and chopped

4 dried apricots, chopped

½ teaspoon grated lemon zest

½ teaspoon ground cinnamon

30 g (1 oz) apricot jam

20 g (¾ oz) butter or margarine

60 ml (2 fl oz) honey

4½ tablespoons (90 ml/3 fl oz) orange juice

½ teaspoon grated nutmeg

CREAMED RICE WITH SLICED PEARS

A yummy variation on creamed rice with an intermediate G.I.

•

G.I. FACTOR: 56
NUTRIENTS PER SERVING: 287 kcal (1250 kJ)

FAT .... neg.
CARBOHYDRATE .... 65 g
FIBRE .... 3 g

500 ml (18 fl oz) water

200 g (7 oz) Basmati rice

185 ml (6 fl oz) evaporated
  skimmed milk

55 g (2 oz) brown sugar

5 ml (1 teaspoon) vanilla essence

420 g (15 oz) can pear slices

1. Bring the water to the boil in a saucepan, add the rice and boil for 15 minutes; drain.

2. Return the rice to the saucepan with the milk. Stir over low heat until all the milk is absorbed. Stir in the sugar and vanilla essence; cool.

3. Using an ice cream scoop, serve scoops of rice with the pear slices.

SERVES 4

CREAMY APRICOT SLICE

To toast coconut, cook in a nonstick frying pan over low heat, stirring for 2 minutes or until just golden. Remove from the pan to cool.

●

G.I. FACTOR: 46

NUTRIENTS PER SERVING: 257 kcal (1080 kJ)

FAT..............................12 g
CARBOHYDRATE..........32 g
FIBRE...........................2 g

1. Line an 18 x 28 cm (7 x 11 inch) rectangular roasting tin with foil.

2. For the base, combine the ingredients in a bowl and mix well. Press the mixture evenly over the base of the prepared tin.

3. Bake in a moderate oven (180°C/350°F/Gas Mark 4) for about 10 minutes or until browned. Remove from oven and allow to cool.

4. For the topping, cover the apricots with the boiling water, and let stand for 30 minutes or until soft. Process in a blender or food processor until smooth. Add the yoghurt, honey and eggs and blend until smooth.

5. Spread the topping mixture over the prepared base. Bake in a moderate oven (180°C/350°F/Gas Mark 4) for about 30 to 35 minutes or until set.

6. Cool, then refrigerate several hours before serving.

SERVES 8

BASE
20 g (¾ oz) desiccated coconut, toasted

125 g (4½ oz) oatmeal biscuits, finely crushed

60 g (2 oz) butter or margarine, melted

TOPPING
125 g (4½ oz) dried apricots

125 ml (4½ fl oz) boiling water

2 x 200 g (14 oz) cartons low-fat apricot yoghurt

60 ml (2 fl oz) honey

2 eggs

REFRESHING FRUIT CHEESECAKE

A delicious lower fat cheesecake that leaves you feeling good after you eat it — not weighed down with fat.

●

G.I. FACTOR: 53
NUTRIENTS PER SERVING: 43 kcal (180 kJ)

FAT	14 g
CARBOHYDRATE	35 g
FIBRE	1 g

BASE

250 g (9 oz) oatmeal biscuits, crushed

90 g (3½ oz) butter or margarine, melted

FILLING

2 teaspoons gelatine

30 ml (2 tablespoons) boiling water

200 g (7 oz) carton low-fat fruit yoghurt

250 g (9 oz) carton low-fat pineapple cottage cheese

60 ml (2 fl oz) honey

2.5 ml (½ teaspoon) vanilla essence

200 g (7 oz) chopped fresh fruit (e.g. apple, orange, cantaloupe melon, strawberries, pear, grapes)

1. For the base, combine the biscuit crumbs and butter in a bowl. Press evenly into a 23 cm (9 inch) pie dish. Bake in a moderate oven (180°C/350°F/ Gas Mark 4) for 10 minutes. Cool.

2. For the filling, sprinkle the gelatine over the boiling water in a cup, stand cup in a small pan of simmering water and stir until dissolved; cool slightly.

3. Process the cooled gelatine with the yoghurt, cottage cheese, honey and vanilla essence in a blender or food processor until smooth.

4. Arrange the chopped fruit over the prepared crust and pour over the yoghurt mixture. Refrigerate for about 1 hour or until set.

SERVES 8

Don't use pawpaw, pineapple or kiwifruit as these tend to prevent gelatine from setting.

YOGHURT BERRY JELLY

An easy dessert. You could make it with low-calorie jelly crystals if you wanted to reduce the energy content.

●

G.I. FACTOR: 54
NUTRIENTS PER SERVING: 86 kcal (360 kJ)

FAT	neg.
CARBOHYDRATE	16 g
FIBRE	1 g

1. Combine the jelly and the boiling water in a bowl, stir until dissolved; cool but do not allow to set.

2. Roughly chop the strawberries (frozen raspberries will tend to break up on stirring).

3. Fold the yoghurt and berries through the jelly; mix well. Pour into serving bowls, cover and refrigerate until set.

SERVES 4

85 g (3 oz) packet berry-flavoured jelly

250 ml (9 fl oz) boiling water

145 g (5 oz) strawberries or frozen raspberries

300 g (10½ oz) low-fat berry yoghurt

FRUIT COMPOTE

*An easily made all-year-round fruity favourite that is especially popular
with children.*

•

G.I. FACTOR: 41
NUTRIENTS PER SERVING: 240 kcal (1030 kJ)

FAT .... 1 g
CARBOHYDRATE .... 65 g
FIBRE .... 10 g

95 g (3½ oz) sultanas

160 g (5½ oz) prunes

190 g (7 oz) dried apricots

175 ml (6 fl oz) orange juice

½ cinnamon stick

1 fresh pear, diced

1. Place the dried fruit, orange juice and
   cinnamon stick in a heavy-bottomed
   saucepan. Bring to the boil, then simmer
   gently for 30 minutes.

2. After 30 minutes, add the diced pear and
   simmer for another 10 minutes. Discard
   the cinnamon and leave the fruit to
   cool.

3. Serve cold with natural yoghurt, or use
   as a topping for porridge.

SERVES 4 TO 6

SNACKS

CHICK PEA AND SESAME PUREE

CHICK NUTS

CURRIED LENTIL SPREAD

CHEESE AND HERB OAT SCONES

SPICY BEAN DIP

LOW-FAT MUESLI BARS

MUESLI MUNCHIES

OAT AND APPLE MUFFINS

APRICOT FLAPJACK

SNACK BARS

●

CHICK PEA AND SESAME PUREE

This spread is a healthy alternative to margarine for sandwiches and crackers but is also delicious eaten alone with Lebanese pitta bread.

•

G.I. FACTOR: 32
NUTRIENTS PER SERVING: 81 kcal (340 kJ)
(1 tablespoon)

FAT ....6 g
CARBOHYDRATE ....4 g
FIBRE ....2 g

140 g (5 oz) dried chick peas

1.5 litres (2½ pt) water

2 cloves garlic, crushed

185 ml (6 fl oz) tahini (sesame seed paste)

½ teaspoon salt

juice of 2 lemons

1 teaspoon ground cumin

1 teaspoon minced chilli

olive oil

ground paprika

chopped fresh parsley

1. Soak the chick peas overnight in the water.

2. Bring the chick peas in some fresh water to the boil in a large saucepan, reduce the heat and simmer for 2 hours.

3. Drain the chick peas and reserve 4 tablespoons of the cooking water. Rinse the chick peas under cold water and drain.

4. Reserve 3 tablespoons of chick peas for garnish and purée the remaining chick peas in a food processor, adding a little of the reserved water if necessary.

5. Combine the chick pea purée, garlic, tahini and salt in a bowl. Add the lemon juice, cumin and chilli; mix well.

6. Spoon into a shallow serving bowl. Serve drizzled with a little olive oil and sprinkled with paprika, parsley and reserved chick peas.

CHICK NUTS

A tasty low-fat, low G.I. nibble. Spice them up with the flavourings suggested or your own combinations. All you need is some chick peas.

●

G.I. FACTOR: 33
100 g (3½ oz) CHICK PEAS PROVIDES: 321 kcal (1350 kJ)

FAT	6 g
CARBOHYDRATE	45 g
FIBRE	15 g

1. Soak the chick peas in water overnight. Next day, drain and pat dry with paper towels.

2. Spread the chick peas in a single layer on a baking tray. Bake in a moderate oven (180°C/350°F/Gas Mark 4) for about 45 minutes or until completely crisp. (They will shrink to their original size.)

3. Toss with a flavouring (see below) while hot, or cool and serve plain.

375 g (13 oz) packet dried chick peas

FLAVOUR VARIATIONS

Chick Devils
Sprinkle a mixture of cayenne pepper and salt over the hot chick nuts.

Red Chicks
Sprinkle a mixture of paprika and garlic salt over the hot chick nuts.

CURRIED LENTIL SPREAD

*A low-fat savoury spread that can be served with
Lebanese pitta bread, pappadums or plain crackers.*

•

G.I. FACTOR: 26
NUTRIENTS PER SERVING: 17 kcal (70 kJ)
(1 tablespoon)

FAT ....1 g
CARBOHYDRATE ....1 g
FIBRE ....0.5 g

125 g (4½ oz) red lentils

about 400 ml (14 fl oz) water

25 g (1 oz) butter or margarine

1 small onion, finely chopped

2 tablespoons curry powder

salt

freshly ground black pepper

1. Combine the lentils and water in a saucepan, bring to the boil, reduce the heat and simmer for about 20 to 30 minutes or until the water is absorbed. Mash with a fork.

2. Melt the butter in a small saucepan, add the onion and cook for about 5 minutes or until soft.

3. Add the curry powder and cook for a further 1 to 2 minutes.

4. Blend or process the lentils and onion mixture to make a smooth paste. Add salt and pepper to taste. Cool before serving.

CHEESE AND HERB OAT SCONES

These savoury scones make a delicious light lunch with salad or a tasty snack on their own. They are ready to eat as they are!

●

G.I. FACTOR: 58

NUTRIENTS PER SCONE: 126 kcal (530 kJ)

FAT	5 g
CARBOHYDRATE	17 g
FIBRE	3 g

1. Sift the flour and baking powder into a large bowl, stir in the oat bran. Rub in the butter or margarine.

2. Make a well in the centre and add the milk and half the water. Mix lightly with a knife, adding extra water if necessary, to make a soft dough. Turn the dough onto a lightly floured board and knead gently.

3. Roll out the dough to a rectangle about 1 cm (½ inch) thick. Scatter half the cheese and all the herbs over the entire surface.

4. Beginning from a long side, roll up like a Swiss roll to make a thick sausage. Cut into 3 cm (1½ inch) slices to make little rounds.

5. Place the rounds side by side on a greased baking tray and sprinkle with the remaining cheese. Bake in a hot oven (200°C/400°F/Gas Mark 6) for about 20 minutes or until golden brown. Serve hot or cold.

150 g (5½ oz) self-raising flour, sifted

1½ teaspoons baking powder

140 g (5 oz) unprocessed oat bran

30 g (1 oz) butter or margarine

125 ml (4½ fl oz) semi-skimmed milk

30 ml (2 tablespoons) water

60 g (2 oz) grated low-fat cheddar cheese

2 teaspoons chopped fresh parsley

2 teaspoons chopped fresh basil or 1 teaspoon dried basil leaves

1 teaspoon dried rosemary leaves

MAKES 10 SCONES

SPICY BEAN DIP

This dip is hot to taste but that's the appeal of it!
Use as a dip with crackers or as a tasty pasta sauce.

•

G.I. FACTOR: 47
NUTRIENTS PER SERVING: 171 kcal (720 kJ)

FAT ....3 g
CARBOHYDRATE..........18 g
FIBRE ....7.3 g

10 ml (2 teaspoons) olive oil

1 medium onion (120 g/4 oz), finely chopped

1 medium green pepper (150 g/ 5½ oz), finely chopped

1 teaspoon curry powder

1 teaspoon minced chilli

10–15 ml (2–3 teaspoons) Worcestershire sauce

420 g (15 oz) can kidney beans, drained

250 ml (9 fl oz) tomato purée

250 ml (9 fl oz) red wine

1. Heat the oil in a nonstick frying pan or small saucepan. Add the onion and green pepper and cook for about 5 minutes or until soft. Add the curry powder and chilli and cook for a further 30 seconds.

2. Stir in the Worcestershire sauce, beans, tomato purée and wine. Bring to the boil.

3. Reduce heat and simmer, uncovered, for about 20 minutes or until thickened.

SERVES 4 AS A SAUCE

LOW-FAT MUESLI BARS

*These bars have a heavy, wholesome texture and make a
very sustaining snack if you are hungry.*

•

G.I. FACTOR: 54
NUTRIENTS PER BAR: 140 kcal (590 kJ)

FAT ....8 g
CARBOHYDRATE..........15 g
FIBRE............................3 g

1. Line a shallow 20 x 30 cm (8 x 12 inch) baking tin with nonstick baking paper.

2. Sift the flours, baking powder and spices into a large bowl. Stir in the oats, fruit and seeds and stir to combine.

3. Add the apple juice, oil and whole egg; mix well. Gently mix in the egg whites until combined.

4. Press the mixture evenly into the prepared tin and press firmly with the back of a spoon. Mark the surface into 12 bars using a sharp knife.

5. Bake in a hot oven (200°C/400°F/Gas Mark 6) for about 15 to 20 minutes or until lightly browned. Cool and cut into bars.

MAKES 12 BARS

75 g (2½ oz) wholemeal plain flour

75 g (2½ oz) self-raising flour

1 teaspoon baking powder

½ teaspoon mixed spice

½ teaspoon ground cinnamon

135 g (5 oz) rolled oats

150 g (5½ oz) dried fruit medley or dried fruit of choice, chopped

35 g (1½ oz) sunflower seed kernels

125 ml (4½ fl oz) apple juice

60 ml (2 fl oz) oil

1 egg, lightly beaten

2 egg whites, lightly beaten

MUESLI MUNCHIES

*Crunchy little bite-sized biscuits which make
handy low G.I. snacks.*

•

G.I. FACTOR: 56
NUTRIENTS PER BISCUIT: 140 kcal (590 kJ)

FAT	8 g
CARBOHYDRATE	15 g
FIBRE	3 g

90 g (3½ oz) butter or margarine

60 ml (2 fl oz) honey

1 egg

*2.5 ml (½ teaspoon) vanilla
essence*

300 g (10½ oz) natural muesli

*2 tablespoons sunflower seed
kernels*

*40 g (1½ oz) self-raising flour,
sifted*

1. Melt the butter and honey in a small saucepan.

2. Whisk the egg and vanilla essence together in a large bowl.

3. Add the butter mixture, muesli, sunflower seed kernels and flour to the egg mixture; stir until combined.

4. Place small spoonfuls of the mixture onto a lightly greased baking tray, spacing evenly.

5. Bake in a moderately hot oven (190°C/ 375°F/Gas Mark 5) for about 10 minutes or until golden brown. Let stand on tray until firm, then loosen and place on a wire rack to cool.

MAKES 16 BISCUITS

OAT AND APPLE MUFFINS

These are delicious low-fat muffins, with
moist chunks of apple through them.

•

G.I. FACTOR: 56
NUTRIENTS PER MUFFIN: 102 kcal (430 kJ)

FAT ....1 g
CARBOHYDRATE..........22 g
FIBRE..........................2 g

1. Combine the All-Bran™ and milk in a bowl and let stand for 10 minutes.

2. Sift the flour, baking powder and mixed spice into a large bowl. Stir in the oat bran, sultanas and apple.

3. Combine the egg, honey and vanilla essence in a bowl. Add the egg mixture and All-Bran™ mixture to the dry ingredients and stir with a wooden spoon until just combined. Do not over-mix.

4. Spoon the mixture into a greased 12-hole muffin tray. Bake in a moderate oven (180°C/350°F/Gas Mark 4) for about 15 minutes or until lightly browned and cooked through. Serve warm or cold.

MAKES 12 MUFFINS

40 g (1½ oz) All-Bran™ cereal

165 ml (6 fl oz) semi-skimmed milk

75 g (2½ oz) self-raising flour

2 teaspoons baking powder

1 teaspoon mixed spice

75 g (2½ oz) unprocessed oat bran

80 g (3 oz) sultanas

1 green apple, peeled and cut into 5 mm (¼ inch) cubes

1 egg, lightly beaten

60 ml (2 fl oz) honey

2.5 ml (½ teaspoon) vanilla essence

If you find them too dry when cold, warm in the microwave (100% power) for 10 seconds before serving.

Warm the honey first to make measuring easy.

APRICOT FLAPJACK

A tasty, chewy snack or light lunch dessert course.

•

G.I. FACTOR: 52
NUTRIENTS PER SERVING: 150 kcal (640 kJ)

FAT ....6 g
CARBOHYDRATE..........21 g
FIBRE...........................2 g

100 g (3½ oz) polyunsaturated
margarine

200 g (7 oz) golden syrup

240 g (8½ oz) jumbo porridge
oats

100 g (3½ oz) no-soak dried
apricots, chopped

1. Lightly grease a shallow 18 x 28 cm (7 x
   11 inch) baking tin.

2. Gently warm the margarine and syrup
   together until the margarine is melted.
   Add the oats and apricots, and stir well
   to combine the ingredients. Tip the
   mixture into the prepared tin and press
   out evenly.

3. Bake in the middle of a moderate oven
   (190°C/375°F/Gas Mark 5) for 20
   minutes or until golden.

4. Remove the tin from the oven and leave
   the flapjack to cool in the tin. When
   cold, cut into 16 portions and store in
   an airtight tin.

MAKES 16 PIECES

SNACK BARS

These filling, chewy bars are ideal for a quick low-fat snack.

•

G.I. FACTOR: 54
NUTRIENTS PER BAR: 160 kcal (672 kJ)

FAT	3 g
CARBOHYDRATE	29 g
FIBRE	3 g

1. Lightly grease a shallow 20 cm (8 inch) square or 18 x 28 cm (7 x 11 inch) rectangular baking tin.

2. Combine all the ingredients thoroughly in a large bowl. Press into the prepared tin and bake in a moderate oven (180°C/350°F/Gas Mark 4) for about 30 minutes until golden brown.

3. Cut into bars while still warm but leave in the tin until cool. Store in an airtight tin.

MAKES 10 PIECES

4 Weetabix™, crumbled

60 g (2 oz) wholemeal self-raising flour

90 g (3 oz) no-soak dried apricots

60 g (2 oz) sultanas

100 g (3½ oz) pitted prunes

15 ml (1 tablespoon) groundnut oil

1 large egg, lightly beaten

60 g (2 oz) caster sugar

125 g (4½ oz) low-fat natural yoghurt

PART III

THE G.I. FACTOR TABLE

HOW TO USE THE G.I. FACTOR TABLE

....

THE G.I. FACTOR TABLE

....

SOURCES AND FURTHER READING

....

HOW TO USE THE
G.I. FACTOR TABLE

•

The following simplified table is an A to Z listing of the G.I. factor of foods commonly eaten. Approximately 250 different foods are listed. They include some new values for foods tested only recently.

The G.I. value shown next to each food is the average for that food using glucose as the standard, i.e. glucose has a G.I. value of 100, with other foods rated accordingly. The average may represent the mean of 10 studies of that food worldwide or only 2 to 4 studies. In a few instances, Australian data are different from the rest of the world and we show Australian data rather than the average. Rice and porridge fall into this category.

We have included some foods in the list which are not commonly eaten (e.g. gram dhal) and other foods which may be encountered on overseas trips.

To check on a food's G.I., simply look for it by name in the alphabetical list. You may also find it under a food type — e.g. fruit, biscuits.

Included in the table is the carbohydrate (CHO) and fat content of a sample serving of the food. This is to help you keep track of the amount of fat and carbohydrate in your diet. Remember, when you are choosing foods, the G.I. factor isn't the only thing to consider. In terms of your blood sugar levels you should also consider the amount of carbohydrate you are eating. For your overall health, the fat, fibre and micronutrient content of your diet is also important. A dietitian can guide you further with good food choices (see page 13).

THE G.I. FACTOR TABLE

A TO Z OF FOODS WITH G.I. FACTOR,

CARBOHYDRATE (CHO) AND FAT

Food	G.I.	Fat	CHO
		\(grams per serving\)	
All Bran™, 40 g	42	1	22
Angel food cake, 30 g	67	trace	17
Apple, 1 medium, 150 g	38	0	18
Apple juice, unsweetened, 250 ml	40	0	33
Apple muffin, 1, 80 g	44	10	44
Apricots, fresh, 3 medium, 100 g	57	0	7
canned, light syrup, 125 g	64	0	13
dried, 5–6 pieces, 30 g	31	0	13
Bagel, 1 white, 70 g	72	1	35
Baked beans, canned in tomato sauce, 120 g	48	1	13
Banana cake, 1 slice, 80 g	47	7	46
Banana, raw, 1 medium, 150 g	55	0	32
Barley, pearled, boiled, 80 g	25	1	17
Basmati white rice, boiled, 180 g	58	0	50
Beetroot, canned, drained, 2–3 slices, 60 g	64	0	5
Bengal gram dhal, 100 g	54	5	57
Biscuits			
Digestives, plain, 2 biscuits, 30 g	59	6	21
Milk Arrowroot, 2 biscuits, 16 g	63	2	13
Morning Coffee, 3 biscuits, 18 g	79	2	14
Oatmeal, 3 biscuits, 30 g	54	6	19
Rich Tea, 2 biscuits, 20 g	55	3	16
Shortbread, 2 biscuits, 30 g	64	8	19
Vanilla wafers, 6 biscuits, 30 g	77	5	21
Wheatmeal, 2 biscuits, 16 g	62	2	12
see also Crackers			
Black bean soup, 220 ml	64	2	82
Black beans, boiled, 120 g	30	1	26
Black gram, soaked and boiled, 120 g	43	1	16
Blackbread, dark rye, 1 slice, 50 g	76	1	21
Blackeyed beans, soaked, boiled, 120 g	42	1	24
Blueberry muffin, 1, 80 g	59	8	41
Bran			
Oat bran, 1 tablespoon, 10 g	55	1	7
Rice bran, extruded, 1 tablespoon, 10 g	19	2	3
Bran Buds™, breakfast cereal, 30 g	58	1	14
Bran muffin, 1, 80 g	60	8	34
Breads			
Dark rye, Blackbread, 1 slice, 50 g	76	1	21
Dark rye, Schinkenbröt, 1 slice, 50 g	86	1	22
French baguette, 30 g	95	1	15
Fruit loaf, heavy, 1 slice, 35 g	47	1	18
Gluten-free bread, 1 slice, 30 g	90	1	14
Hamburger bun, 1 prepacked bun, 50 g	61	3	24
Light rye, 1 slice, 50 g	68	1	23
Linseed rye, 1 slice, 50 g	55	5	21
Melba toast, 4 squares, 30 g	70	1	19
Pitta bread, 1 piece, 65 g	57	1	38

Food	G.I.	Fat	CHO
		(grams per serving)	
Breads (continued)			
Pumpernickel, 2 slices	41	2	35
Rye bread, 1 slice, 50 g	65	1	23
Sourdough rye, 1 slice, 50 g	57	2	23
Vogel's™ Honey & Oat loaf, 1 slice, 40 g	55	3	17
White (wheat flour), 1 slice, 30 g	70	1	15
Wholemeal (wheat flour), 1 slice, 35 g	69	1	14
Bread stuffing, 60 g	74	5	17
Breadfruit, 120 g	68	1	17
Breakfast cereals			
All-Bran™, 40 g	42	1	22
Bran Buds™, 30 g	58	1	14
Cheerios™, 30 g	74	2	20
Coco Pops™, 30 g	77	0	26
Cornflakes, 30 g	84	0	26
Mini Wheats™ (whole wheat), 30 g	58	0	21
Muesli, toasted, 60 g	43	9	33
Muesli, non-toasted, 60 g	56	6	32
Oat bran, raw, 1 tablespoon, 10 g	55	1	7
Porridge (cooked with water), 245 g	42	2	24
Puffed wheat, 30 g	80	1	22
Rice bran, 1 tablespoon, 10 g	19	2	3
Rice Krispies™, 30 g	82	0	27
Shredded wheat, 25 g	67	0	18
Special K™, 30 g	54	0	21
Sultana Bran™, 45 g	52	1	35
Sustain™, 30 g	68	1	25
Weetabix™, 2 biscuits, 30 g	69	1	19
Broad beans, frozen, boiled, 80 g	79	1	9
Buckwheat, cooked, 80 g	54	3	57
Bun, hamburger, 1 prepacked bun, 50 g	61	3	24
Burghul, cooked, 120 g	48	0	22
Butter beans, boiled, 70 g	31	0	13
Cakes			
Angel food cake, 1 slice, 30 g	67	trace	17
Banana cake, 1 slice, 80 g	47	7	46
Flan, 1 slice, 80 g	65	5	55
Pound cake, 1 slice, 80 g	54	15	42
Sponge cake, 1 slice, 60 g	46	16	32
Cantaloupe melon, raw, ¼ small, 200 g	65	0	6
Capellini pasta, boiled, 180 g	45	0	53
Carrots, peeled, boiled, 70 g	49	0	3
Cereal grains			
Barley, pearled, boiled, 80 g	25	1	17
Buckwheat, cooked, 80 g	54	3	57
Burghul, cooked, 120 g	48	0	22
Couscous, cooked, 120 g	65	0	28

Food	G.I.	Fat	CHO
		(grams per serving)	
Cereal grains (continued)			
Maize			
Cornmeal, wholegrain, cooked, 40 g	68	1	30
Sweet corn, canned, drained, 80 g	55	1	16
Taco shells, 2 shells, 26 g	68	6	16
Millet Ragi, cooked, 120 g	71	0	12
Rice			
Basmati, white, boiled, 180 g	58	0	50
Tapioca (boiled with milk), 250 g	81	10.5	51
Cheerios™, breakfast cereal, 30 g	74	2	20
Cherries, 20, 80 g	22	0	10
Chick peas, canned, drained, 95 g	42	2	15
Chick peas, boiled, 120 g	33	3	22
Chocolate, milk, 6 squares, 30 g	49	8	19
Coco Pops™, breakfast cereal, 30 g	77	0	26
Condensed milk, sweetened, ½ cup, 163 g	61	15	90
Corn bran, breakfast cereal, 30 g	75	1	20
Corn chips, Doritos™ original, 50 g	42	11	33
Cornflakes, breakfast cereal, 30 g	84	0	26
Cornmeal (maizemeal), cooked, 40 g	68	1	30
Couscous, cooked, 120 g	65	0	28
Crackers			
Premium soda crackers, 3 biscuits, 25 g	74	4	17
Puffed crispbread, 4 biscuits, wholemeal, 20 g	81	1	15
Rice cakes, 2 cakes, 25 g	82	1	21
Ryvita™, 2 slices, 20 g	69	1	16
Stoned wheat thins, 5 biscuits, 25 g	67	2	17
Water biscuits, 5, 25 g	78	2	18
Croissant, 1	67	14	27
Crumpet, 1, toasted, 50 g	69	0	22
Custard, 175 g	43	5	24
Dairy foods			
Ice cream, full fat, 2 scoops, 50 g	61	6	10
Ice cream, low fat, 2 scoops, 50 g	50	2	13
Milk, full fat, 250 ml	27	10	12
Milk, skimmed, 250 ml	32	0	13
Milk, chocolate flavoured, low-fat, 250 ml	34	3	23
Custard, 175 g	43	5	24
Yoghurt			
low-fat, fruit, 200 g	33	0	26
low-fat, artificial sweetener, 200 g	14	0	12
Dark rye bread, Blackbird, 1 slice, 50 g	76	1	21
Dark rye bread, Schinkenbröt, 1 slice, 50 g	86	1	22
Digestive biscuits, 2 plain, 30 g	59	6	21
Doughnut with cinnamon and sugar, 40 g	76	8	16
Fanta™, soft drink, 1 can, 375 ml	68	0	51
Fettucini, cooked, 180 g	32	1	57

Food	G.I.	Fat	CHO
		(grams per serving)	
Fish fingers, oven-cooked, 5 x 25 g fingers, 125 g	38	14	24
Flan cake, 1 slice, 80 g	65	5	55
French baguette bread, 30 g	95	1	15
French fries, fine cut, small serving, 120 g	75	26	49
Fructose, pure, 10 g	23	0	10
Fruit cocktail, canned in natural juice, 125 g	55	0	15
Fruit loaf, heavy, 1 slice, 35 g	47	1	18
Fruits and fruit products			
Apple, 1 medium, 150 g	38	0	18
Apple juice, unsweetened, 250 ml	40	0	33
Apricots, fresh, 3 medium, 100 g	57	0	7
canned, light syrup, 125 g	64	0	13
dried, 5–6 pieces, 30 g	31	0	13
Banana, raw, 1 medium, 150 g	55	0	32
Cantaloupe melon, raw, ¼ small, 200 g	65	0	10
Cherries, 20, 80 g	22	0	10
Fruit cocktail, canned in natural juice, 125 g	55	0	15
Grapefruit juice, unsweetened, 250 ml	48	0	16
Grapefruit, raw, ½ medium, 100 g	25	0	5
Grapes, green, 100 g	46	0	15
Kiwifruit, 1 raw, peeled, 80 g	52	0	8
Lychee, canned and drained, 7, 90 g	79	0	16
Mango, 1 small, 150 g	55	0	19
Orange, 1 medium, 130 g	44	0	10
Orange juice, 250 ml	46	0	21
Pawpaw, ½ small, 200 g	58	0	14
Peach, fresh, 1 large, 110 g	42	0	7
canned, natural juice, 125 g	30	0	12
canned, heavy syrup, 125 g	58	0	19
canned, light syrup, 125 g	52	0	18
Pear, fresh, 1 medium, 150 g	38	0	21
canned in pear juice, 125 g	44	0	13
Pineapple, fresh, 2 slices, 125 g	66	0	10
Pineapple juice, unsweetened, canned, 250 ml	46	0	27
Plums, 3–4 small, 100 g	39	0	7
Raisins, 40 g	64	0	28
Sultanas, 40 g	56	0	30
Watermelon, 150 g	72	0	8
Gluten-free bread, 1 slice, 30 g	90	1	14
Glutinous rice, white, steamed, 1 cup, 174 g	98	0	37
Gnocchi, cooked, 145 g	68	3	71
Grapefruit juice, unsweetened, 250 ml	48	0	16
Grapefruit, raw, ½ medium, 100 g	25	0	5
Grape Nuts™ cereal, ½ cup, 58 g	71	1	47
Grapes, green, 100 g	46	0	15
Green gram dhal, 100 g	62	4	10
Green gram, soaked and boiled, 120 g	38	1	18

Food	G.I.	Fat	CHO
		(grams per serving)	
Green pea soup, canned, ready to serve, 220 ml	66	1	22
Hamburger bun, 1 prepacked, 50 g	61	3	24
Haricot (navy beans), boiled, 90 g	38	0	11
Honey & Oat Bread (Vogel's™), 1 slice, 40 g	55	3	17
Honey, 1 tablespoon, 20 g	58	0	16
Ice cream, full fat, 2 scoops, 50 g	61	6	10
Ice cream, low-fat, 2 scoops, 50 g	50	2	13
Jelly beans, 5, 10 g	80	0	9
Kidney beans, boiled, 90 g	27	0	18
Kidney beans, canned and drained, 95 g	52	0	13
Kiwifruit, 1 raw, peeled, 80 g	52	0	8
Lactose, pure, 10 g	46	0	10
Lentil soup, canned, 220 ml	44	0	14
Lentils, green and brown, dried, boiled, 95 g	30	0	16
Lentils, red, boiled, 120 g	26	1	21
Light rye bread, 1 slice, 50 g	68	1	23
Linguine pasta, thick, cooked, 180 g	46	1	56
Linguine pasta, thin, cooked, 180 g	55	1	56
Linseed rye bread, 1 slice, 50 g	55	5	21
Lucozade™, original, 1 bottle, 300 ml	95	<1	56
Lungkow bean thread, 180 g	26	0	61
Lychee, canned and drained, 7, 90 g	79	0	16
Macaroni cheese, packaged, cooked, 220 g	64	24	30
Macaroni, cooked, 180 g	45	1	56
Maize			
Cornmeal, wholegrain, 40 g	68	1	30
Sweet corn, canned and drained, 80 g	55	1	16
Maltose (maltodextrins), pure, 10 g	105	0	10
Mango, 1 small, 150 g	55	0	19
Mars Bar™, 60 g	68	11	41
Melba toast, 4 squares, 30 g	70	1	19
Milk, full fat, 250 ml	27	10	12
Milk, skimmed, 250 ml	32	0	13
chocolate flavoured, 250 ml	34	3	23
Milk, sweetened condensed, ½ cup, 160 g	61	15	90
Milk Arrowroot biscuits, 2, 16 g	63	2	13
Millet, cooked, 120 g	71	0	12
Mini Wheats™ (whole wheat) breakfast cereal, 30 g	58	0	21
Morning Coffee biscuits, 3, 18 g	79	2	14
Muesli bars with fruit, 30 g	61	4	17
Muesli, breakfast cereal			
toasted, 60 g	43	9	33
non-toasted, 60 g	56	6	32
Muffins			
Apple, 1 muffin, 80 g	44	10	44
Bran, 1 muffin, 80 g	60	8	34
Blueberry, 1 muffin, 80 g	59	8	41

Food	G.I.	Fat	CHO
		(grams per serving)	
Mung bean noodles, 1 cup, 140 g	39	0	35
Noodles, 2-minute, 85 g packet, cooked	46	16	55
Noodles, rice, fresh, boiled, 1 cup, 176 g	40	0	44
Oat bran, raw, 1 tablespoon, 10 g	55	1	7
Oatmeal biscuits, 3 biscuits, 30 g	54	6	19
Orange, 1 medium, 130 g	44	0	10
Orange juice, 250 ml	46	0	21
Orange squash, diluted, 250 ml	66	0	20
Parsnips, boiled, 75 g	97	0	8
Pasta			
Capellini, cooked, 180 g	45	0	53
Fettucini, cooked, 180 g	32	1	57
Gnocchi, cooked, 145 g	68	3	71
Noodles, 2-minute, 85 g packet, cooked	46	16	55
Linguine, thick, cooked, 180 g	46	1	56
Linguine, thin, cooked, 180 g	55	1	56
Macaroni cheese, packaged, cooked, 220 g	64	24	30
Macaroni, cooked, 180 g	45	1	56
Noodles, mung bean, 1 cup, 140 g	39	0	35
Noodles, rice, fresh, boiled, 1 cup, 176 g	40	0	44
Ravioli, meat-filled, cooked, 220 g	39	11	30
Rice pasta, brown, cooked, 180 g	92	2	57
Spaghetti, white, cooked, 180 g	41	1	56
Spaghetti, wholemeal, cooked, 180 g	37	1	48
Spirale, durum, cooked, 180 g	43	1	56
Star pastina, cooked, 180 g	38	1	56
Tortellini, cheese, cooked, 180 g	50	8	21
Vermicelli, cooked, 180 g	35	0	45
Pastry, flaky, 65 g	59	26	25
Pawpaw, raw, ½ small, 200 g	58	0	14
Pea and ham soup, canned, 220 ml	66	2	13
Peach, fresh, 1 large, 110 g	42	0	7
canned, natural juice, 125 g	30	0	12
canned, heavy syrup, 125 g	58	0	19
canned, light syrup, 125 g	52	0	18
Peanuts, roasted, salted, 75 g	14	40	11
Pear, fresh, 1 medium, 150 g	38	0	21
canned in pear juice, 125 g	44	0	13
Peas, green, fresh, frozen, boiled, 80 g	48	0	5
Peas, dried, boiled, 70 g	22	0	4
Pineapple, fresh, 2 slices, 125 g	66	0	10
Pineapple juice, unsweetened, canned, 250 g	46	0	27
Pinto beans, canned, 95 g	45	0	13
Pinto beans, soaked, boiled, 90 g	39	0	20
Pitta bread, 1 piece, 65 g	57	1	38
Pizza, cheese and tomato, 2 slices, 230 g	60	27	57
Plums, 3–4 small, 100 g	39	0	7
Popcorn, low-fat (popped), 20 g	55	2	10

Food	G.I.	Fat	CHO
		(grams per serving)	
Porridge (made with water), 245 g	42	2	24
Potatoes			
French Fries, fine cut, small serving, 120 g	75	26	49
instant potato	83	1	18
new, peeled, boiled, 5 small (cocktail), 175 g	62	0	23
new, canned, drained, 5 small, 175 g	61	0	20
pale skin, peeled, boiled, 1 medium, 120 g	56	0	16
pale skin, baked in oven (no fat), 1 medium, 120 g	85	0	14
pale skin, mashed, 120 g	70	0	16
pale skin, steamed, 1 medium, 120 g	65	0	17
pale skin, microwaved, 1 medium, 120 g	82	0	17
potato crisps, plain, 50 g	54	16	24
Potato crisps, plain, 50 g	54	16	24
Pound cake, 1 slice, 80 g	54	15	42
Pretzels, 50 g	83	1	22
Puffed crispbread, 4 wholemeal, 20 g	81	1	15
Puffed wheat breakfast cereal, 30 g	80	1	22
Pumpernickel bread, 2 slices	41	2	35
Pumpkin, peeled, boiled, 85 g	75	0	6
Raisins, 40 g	64	0	28
Ravioli, meat-filled, cooked, 220 g	39	11	30
Rice			
Basmati, white, boiled, 180 g	58	0	50
Glutinous, white, steamed, 1 cup, 174 g	98	0	37
Instant, cooked, 180 g	87	0	38
Rice bran, extruded, 1 tablespoon, 10 g	19	2	3
Rice cakes, 2, 25 g	82	1	21
Rice Krispies™, breakfast cereal, 30 g	82	0	27
Rice noodles, fresh, boiled, 1 cup, 176 g	40	0	44
Rice pasta, brown, cooked, 180 g	92	2	57
Rice vermicelli, cooked, 180 g	58	0	58
Rich Tea biscuits, 2, 20 g	55	3	16
Rye bread, 1 slice, 50 g	65	1	23
Ryvita™ crackers, 2 biscuits, 20 g	69	1	16
Sausages, fried, 2, 120 g	28	21	6
Semolina, cooked, 230 g	55	0	17
Shortbread, 2 biscuits, 30 g	64	8	19
Shredded wheat breakfast cereal, 25 g	67	0	18
Soda crackers, 3 biscuits, 25 g	74	4	17
Soft drink, Coca Cola™, 1 can, 375 ml	63	0	40
Soft drink, Fanta™, 1 can, 375 ml	68	0	51
Soups			
Black bean soup, 220 ml	64	2	82
Green pea soup, canned, ready to serve, 220 ml	66	1	22
Lentil soup, canned, 220 ml	44	0	14
Pea and ham soup, 220 ml	60	2	13
Tomato soup, canned, 220 ml	38	1	15
Sourdough rye bread, 1 slice, 50 g	57	2	23

Food	G.I.	Fat	CHO
		(grams per serving)	
Soya beans, canned, 100 g	14	6	12
Soya beans, boiled, 90 g	18	7	10
Spaghetti, white, cooked, 180 g	41	1	56
Spaghetti, wholemeal, cooked, 180 g	37	1	48
Special K™, 30 g	54	0	21
Spirale pasta, durum, cooked, 180 g	43	1	56
Split pea soup, 220 ml	60	0	6
Split peas, yellow, boiled, 90 g	32	0	16
Sponge cake plain, 1 slice, 60 g	46	16	32
Sports drinks			
Gatorade, 250 ml	78	0	15
Isostar, 250ml	70	0	18
Stoned wheat thins, crackers, 5 biscuits, 25 g	67	2	17
Sucrose, 1 teaspoon	65	0	5
Sultana Bran™, 45 g	52	1	35
Sultanas, 40 g	56	0	30
Sustain™, 30 g	68	1	25
Swede, peeled, boiled, 60 g	72	0	3
Sweet corn, 85 g	55	1	16
Sweet potato, peeled, boiled, 80 g	54	0	16
Sweetened condensed milk, ½ cup, 160 g	61	15	90
Taco shells, 2, 26 g	68	6	16
Tapioca pudding, boiled with milk, 250 g	81	10.5	51
Tapioca, steamed 1 hour, 100 g	70	6	54
Tofu frozen dessert (non-dairy), 100 g	115	1	13
Tomato soup, canned, 220 ml	38	1	15
Tortellini, cheese, cooked, 180 g	50	8	21
Vanilla wafer biscuits, 6, 30 g	77	5	21
Vermicelli, cooked, 180 g	35	0	45
Waffles, 25 g	76	3	9
Water biscuits, 5, 25 g	78	2	18
Watermelon, 150 g	72	0	8
Weetabix™ breakfast cereal, 2 biscuits, 30 g	69	1	19
Wheatmeal biscuits, 2, 16 g	62	2	12
White bread, wheat flour, 1 slice, 30 g	70	1	15
Wholemeal bread, wheat flour, 1 slice, 35 g	69	1	14
Yakult, 65 ml serve	46	0	11
Yam, boiled, 80 g	51	0	26
Yoghurt			
low-fat, fruit, 200 g	33	0	26
low-fat, artificial sweetener, 200 g	14	0	12

■■■ SOURCES AND FURTHER READING

Behall KM, Schofield DJ, Canary J. Effect of starch structure on glucose and insulin responses in human subjects. Am J Clin Nutr, 1988, 47 : 428–32

Brand JC, Colagiuri S, Crossman S, Allen A, Roberts DCK, Truswell AS. Low glycemic index foods improve long term glycemic control in NIDDM. Diabetes Care, 1991, 14 : 95–101

Brand JC, Nicholson PL, Thorburn AW, Truswell AS. Food processing and the glycemic index. Am J Clin Nutr, 1985, 42 : 1192–6

Brand Miller J. The importance of glycemic index in diabetes. Am J Clin Nutr, 1994, 59 (suppl) : 747s–752s

Brand Miller J, Colagiuri S. The carnivore connection: dietary carbohydrate in the evolution of non-insulin dependent diabetes. Diabetologia, 1994, 37 : 1280–6

Brand Miller J, Lobbezoo I. Replacing starch with sucrose in a high glycaemic index breakfast cereal lowers glycaemic and insulin responses. Eur J Clin Nutr, 1994, 48 : 749–502

Brand Miller J, Pang E, Bramall L. Rice: a high or low glycemic index food? Am J Clin Nutr, 1992, 56 : 1034–6

Brand Miller J, Pang E, Broomhead L. The glycemic index of foods containing sugars: comparison of foods with naturally occurring versus added sugars. Brit J Nutr, 1995, 73 : 613–23

Burke L, Collier G, Hargreaves M. Muscle glycogen storage following prolonged exercise: effect of the glycaemic index of carbohydrate feedings. J Appl Physiol, 1993, 74 : 1019–23

Burke LM, *The Complete Guide to Food for Sports Performance*. Allen & Unwin, 1992

Byrnes S, Denyer G, Brand Miller J, Storlein L. The effect of amylose vs amylopectin feeding on development of insulin resistance in rats. J Nutr, 1995, 125 : 1430–7

Coyle EF. Substrate utilisation during exercise in active people. Am J Clin Nutr, 1995, 61 : 968S–979S

Coyle EF. Timing and method of increased carbohydrate intake to cope with heavy training, competition and recovery. J Sport Sci, 1991, 9 spec : 29–51

Foster-Powell K, Brand Miller J. International tables of glycemic index. Am J Clin Nutr, 1995, 62 : 871S–893S

Frost G, Keogh B, Smith D, Akinsanya K, Leeds A. Effect of a low glycaemic index diet on insulin and glucose response in vitro and in vivo in patients with coronary heart disease. Metabolism, 1996, 45 (6) : 669–72

Frost, G, Keogh B, Smith D, Leeds AR. Differences in glucose uptake in adipocytes from patients with and without coronary heart disease. Diabetic Medicine, 1998, 15 : 1003–9

Frost G, Leeds AR, Dore CJB, Madieros S, Brading SA, Dornhorst A. Glycaemic index as a determinant of serum high density lipoprotein. Lancet, 1999, 353 : 1045–8

Frost G, Trew G, Margara R, Leeds A, Dornhurst A. The effect of low glycaemic index carbohydrate on insulin sensitivity in women with a family history of heart disease. Diabetologia, 1997, 40, Supplement 1 A338 (1528)

Frost G, Wilding J, Beecham J. Dietary advice based on the glycaemic advice improves dietary profile and metabolic control in Type 2 diabetic patients. Diabetic Medicine, 1994, 11 : 397–401

Grandfeldt Y, Bjork I, Hagander B. On the importance of processing conditions, product thickness and egg addition for the glycaemic and hormonal responses to pasta: a comparison with bread made from 'pasta ingredients'. Eur J Clin Nutr, 1991, 45 : 489–99

Heaton KW, Marcus SN, Emmett PM, Bolton CH. Particle size of wheat, maize, and oat test meals: effects on plasma glucose and insulin responses and on the rate of starch digestion in vitro. Am J Clin Nutr, 1988, 47 : 675–82

Holt S, Brand JC, Soveny C, Hansky J. Relationship of satiety to postprandial glycaemic, insulin and cholescystokinin responses. Appetite, 1992, 18 : 129–41

Holt S, Brand Miller J. Particle size, satiety and the glycaemic response. Eur J Clin Nutr, 1994, 48 : 496–502

Inge K and Brukner P. *Food for Sport*. William Heinemann, 1986

Jenkins DJA, Wolever TMS, Taylor RH, et al. Glycaemic index of foods: a physiological basis for carbohydrate exchange. Am J Clin Nutr, 1981, 34 : 362–6

Lingstrom P, Holm J, Birkhed D, Bjorck I. Effects of variously processed starch on pH of human dental plaque. Scan J Dent Res, 1989, 97 : 392–400

Liu S, Stampfer MJ, Manson JE, Hu FB, Franz M, Hennekens CH, Willet WC. A prospective study of dietary glycaemic load and risk of myocardial infarction in women. FASEB, 1998, 124 : A260 (abstract #1517)

O'Connor H and Hay D. *The Taste of Fitness*. JB Fairfax Press, 1996

O'Dea K, Nestel PJ, Antonoff L. Physical factors influencing post prandial glucose and insulin responses. Am J Clin Nutr, 1980, 33 : 760–5

Ross SW, Brand JC, Thorburn AW, Truswell AS. Glycemic index of processed wheat products. Am J Clin Nutr, 1987, 46 : 631–5

Salmeron J, Ascherio EB, Rimm GA, Colditz D, Spiegelman D, Jenkins DJ, Stampfer MJ, Wing AL, Willet WC. Dietary fiber, glycaemic load and risk of NIDDM in men. Diabetes Care, 1997, 20 : 545–50

Salmeron J, Manson JE, Stampfer MJ, Colditz GA, Wing AL, Willet WC. Dietary fiber, glycemic load and risk of non-insulin-dependent diabetes mellitus in women. JAMA 1997, 277, 472–7

Slabber M, Barnard HC, Kuyl JM, Dannhauser A, Schall R. Effects of a low-insulin-response, energy-restricted diet on weight loss and plasma insulin concentration in hyper insulinemic obese females. Am J Clin Nutr, 1994, 60 : 48–53

Thomas DE, Brotherhood JR, Brand JC. Carbohydrate feeding before exercise: effect of glycemic index. Internat J Sports Med, 1991, 12 : 180–6

Truswell AS. Glycaemic index of foods. Eur J Clin Nutr, 1992, 46 : S91–S101

Wolever TMS, Jenkins DJA, Jenkins AL, Josse RG. The glycemic index: methodology and clinical implications. Am J Clin Nutr, 1991, 54 : 846–54

Wolever TMS, Nguyen P, Chiasson J, Hunt JA, Josse RG, Palmason C, Rodger NW, Ross SA, Ryan EA, Tan MH. Determinants of diet glycemic index calculated retrospectively from diet records of 342 individuals with non-insulin-dependent diabetes mellitus. Am J Clin Nutr, 1994, 59 : 1265–9

INDEX

■■■■ RECIPE INDEX

DR STEPHEN COLAGIURI, KAYE FOSTER-POWELL, DR JENNIE BRAND MILLER

THE POCKET GUIDE TO THE GLUCOSE REVOLUTION FOR PEOPLE WITH DIABETES

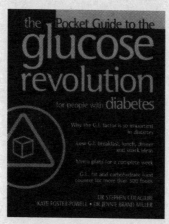

Understanding the G.I. factor has made an enormous difference to the diet and lifestyle of people with diabetes.

Research on the G.I. factor shows that different carbohydrate foods have dramatically different effects on blood sugar levels.

Findings reveal that:
- Many traditionally 'taboo' foods do not cause unfavourable effects on blood sugar.
- Diets with a low G.I. improve blood sugar control in people with diabetes.

The Glucose Revolution for People with Diabetes gives practical advice on how to make the G.I. factor work for you, with tips on meal preparation, a week of low G.I. menus and a table of 300 foods and their nutritional value. Based on the latest scientific research and on the real experiences of real people, it will be an indispensable pocket guide for people with diabetes.

HODDER AND STOUGHTON PAPERBACKS

**KAYE FOSTER-POWELL, DR JENNIE BRAND MILLER,
DR ANTHONY LEEDS**

**THE POCKET GUIDE TO THE GLUCOSE REVOLUTION
AND YOUR HEART**

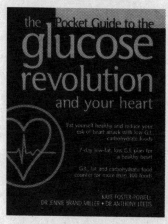

Eat yourself healthy and reduce your risk of heart disease with low-fat (low saturated fat), high-carbohydrate, high-fibre and low G.I. foods.

The latest medical research clearly confirms that slowly digested low G.I. carbohydrate foods like pastas, grainy breads, breakfast cereals based on wheat bran and oats, and many popular Mediterranean-style foods play an important part in treating and preventing heart disease.

What is more, these foods are also important for blood sugar control and weight loss.

This handy pocket guide from the authors of the bestselling *The Glucose Revolution* shows you how to choose the right amount and the right kind of carbohydrate foods for lifelong health and well-being and for reducing the risk of heart attack.

It includes:
- A 7-day low-fat, low G.I. meal plan for heart health.
- The low-fat, low G.I. healthy heart pantry checklist.
- G.I. factor, fat and carbohydrate content of more than 300 tested foods.

HODDER AND STOUGHTON PAPERBACKS

**KAYE FOSTER-POWELL, DR JENNIE BRAND MILLER,
DR STEPHEN COLAGIURI**

**THE POCKET GUIDE TO THE GLUCOSE REVOLUTION
AND LOSING WEIGHT**

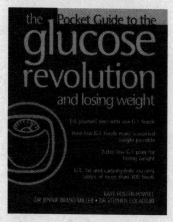

Eating to lose weight is easy with low G.I. foods because you do
not have to go hungry.

Not all foods are created equal when it comes to losing weight.
The latest medical research shows that low G.I. carbohydrate
foods have special advantages because they fill you up and keep
you satisfied for longer.

Carbohydrates are natural appetite suppressants, and of all
carbohydrate foods, those with a low G.I. factor prevent hunger
pangs longer without providing excess kilojoules.

This pocket guide will help you eat yourself slim with low G.I.
foods and includes:
- A 7-day G.I. plan for losing weight.
- G.I. factor, fat content and carbohydrate content tables of
  more than 300 tested foods.

HODDER AND STOUGHTON PAPERBACKS

**DR HELEN O'CONNOR, DR JENNIE BRAND MILLER,
DR STEPHEN COLAGIURI, KAYE FOSTER-POWELL**

**THE POCKET GUIDE TO THE GLUCOSE REVOLUTION
AND SPORTS NUTRITION**

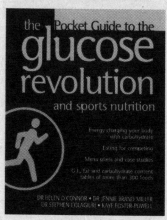

Whether you are a serious athlete or a weekend warrior, what you eat can make a big difference to your performance. Carbohydrates are the key. Manipulating the G.I. of your diet can give you the winning edge.

The Pocket Guide to the Glucose Revolution and Sports Nutrition shows how high carbohydrate diets enhance stamina and prevent fatigue. It is filled with fun, easy and practical suggestions and is ideal for sports people, gymnasts and dancers who want to eat their way to better performance.

HODDER AND STOUGHTON PAPERBACKS